HIKES LIST

MENASHA RIDGE PRESS
Birmingham, Alabama

60 HIKES WITHIN 60 MILES

SALT LAKE CITY

INCLUDING
**Ogden, Provo,
and the Uintas**

SECOND EDITION

GREG WITT

60 HIKES WITHIN 60 MILES: SALT LAKE CITY

Copyright © 2012 Greg Witt
All rights reserved
Printed in the United States of America
Published by Menasha Ridge Press
Distributed by Publishers Group West
Second edition, first printing

Library of Congress Cataloging-in-Publication Data

Witt, Greg, 1952–
    60 hikes within 60 miles Salt Lake City : including Ogden, Provo,
    and the Uintas / Greg Witt. — 2nd ed.
        p. cm.
    Includes index.
    ISBN-13: 978-0-89732-942-2
    ISBN-10: 0-89732-942-2
    1. Hiking—Utah—Salt Lake City Region—Guidebooks. 2. Salt Lake
    City Region (Utah)—Guidebooks. I. Title.
    GV199.42.U73W58 2012
    917.92—dc23

                                                2012014902

Editor: Ritchey Halphen
Cover design: Scott McGrew
Cartography and elevation profiles: Scott McGrew and Greg Witt
Text design: Steveco International
Cover photo: Rob Witt
Interior photos: Greg Witt except as noted on-page
Proofreader: Susan Roberts
Indexer: Jan Mucciarone/Elite Editorial Services

Menasha Ridge Press
P.O. Box 43673
Birmingham, Alabama 35243
menasharidge.com

DISCLAIMER

This book is meant only as a guide to select trails in the Salt Lake City area and does not guarantee hiker safety—you hike at your own risk. Neither Menasha Ridge Press nor Greg Witt is liable in any way for property loss or damage, personal injury, or death that result from accessing or hiking the trails described in the following pages. Be especially cautious when walking on or near boulders, steep inclines, and drop-offs, and do not explore terrain that may be beyond your abilities. To help ensure an uneventful hike, carefully read the introduction to this book and get further safety information and guidance from other sources. Familiarize yourself with current weather reports, maps of the area you intend to visit (in addition to the maps in this guidebook), and any relevant park regulations. While every effort has been made to ensure the accuracy of this guidebook, land and road conditions, phone numbers and websites, and other information can change from year to year.

TABLE OF CONTENTS

ACKNOWLEDGMENTS

A PROJECT OF THIS MAGNITUDE goes from concept to print with the contributions of many. I'm thankful for the energetic and talented team at Menasha Ridge Press, who approached me about writing a Salt Lake City hiking guide. I was somewhat reluctant at first, but through their encouragement, vision, and support, *60 Hikes* became a reality.

Thanks to Sheryl McGlochlin, whose energy and enthusiasm are infectious. She's introduced many of these hikes to hundreds of locals and is always anxious to share a favorite hike with friends like me.

I'm appreciative of the staff at Weber Pathways, who have created a hiking legacy for the Ogden area through their efforts to promote, plan, and preserve trails.

I'm grateful to Alan and Kristine Colledge, with whom I've shared gallons of Gatorade and miles of terrain across the Wasatch, the Colorado Plateau, and the Grand Canyon.

Thanks to my parents, Bud and Claire Witt, who took me on hikes in Mill Creek Canyon and Brighton as a toddler. Later, they led me to discover the Sierra Nevada and many national parks on fabulous cross-country road trips.

I've met hundreds of hikers along the trail. Sometimes our exchange was nothing more than "g'morning" or "hello." But often these newfound friends would share their experiences with me—identifying a wildflower, reporting on a moose sighting, or telling me about a favorite waterfall just up the canyon. Their insights and love of the outdoors have enriched my life and are woven into every hike in this book.

Many of those trail acquaintances were members of the Wasatch Mountain Club, an organization of dedicated volunteers who love to explore the scenic wonders of the area mountains. They also deserve much of the credit for improving the quality of the outdoor experience through preservation of wild lands and providing access to these pristine reaches.

Special thanks to many hiking friends who have provided ideas, encouragement, and support along the way, including Phil Schow, Mark McGuire, Bart Hamatake, Bruce Bown, Ben Adcock, Peter Tennis, David Crowther, Jim Rasband, Vaughn Armstrong, Jim McDonald, Mary Baxter, Jack Welch, Al Christy, Jim Driggs, Harlan Hatfield, and Dennis Hoagland.

I always cherish the time I've spent on these and other Utah trails with my children, Heather, Blair, Lindsey, Dallin, and Tessa. I look forward to sharing many more trail miles with my grandchildren, Hannah, Isaac, Alden, and Grant.

My deepest gratitude goes to my wife, Elain, my best friend and eternal trail companion. Her sustaining belief, encouragement, and love have guided me through this project and every other aspect of my life. She joined me on many of these hikes, but I wish she could have joined me on every one. If she had, this would have been a far more elaborate book.

—*Greg Witt*

ABOUT THE AUTHOR

GREG WITT has lived the adventures he writes about and shares with audiences around the world. His journeys have taken him to every corner of the globe. He has guided mountaineering expeditions in the Alps and Andes and paddled wild rivers in the Americas. He has dropped teams of adventurers into golden slot canyons; trudged through deep jungles in Africa, Central America, and Asia; and guided archaeological expeditions across the parched Arabian Peninsula.

After earning degrees from the University of California and Brigham Young University, Greg had an early career in human-resources management. But because he prefers high adventure to the high-rise, he traded his wingtips for hiking boots decades ago and has never looked back.

Some weeks, Greg hikes more miles than he drives, which means he wears out his boots faster than he wears out his tires. He has crossed the Grand Canyon on foot more than a dozen times and climbed Colorado's three highest peaks in three days. Each summer in the Swiss Alps, he hikes more than 700 miles and gains nearly 100,000 vertical feet of elevation as he guides guests of Alpenwild, a company he owns and operates.

Greg loves leading readers on the most breathtaking hikes and exciting outdoor adventures on the globe. He comes ready to discuss the geology, history, archaeology, weather patterns, culture, flora, and fauna of the exciting locales he loves. His other books include *Exploring Havasupai* (Menasha Ridge Press), *Ultimate Adventures: A Rough Guide to Adventure Travel* (Rough Guides), and the forthcoming *50 Best Short Hikes: Salt Lake City* (Wilderness Press).

Greg's research and exploration continue to uncover surprising adventures just waiting to be experienced. If you join him, you'll be guaranteed a phenomenal journey.

FOREWORD

WELCOME TO MENASHA RIDGE PRESS'S *60 Hikes within 60 Miles,* a series designed to provide hikers with the information they need to find and hike the very best trails surrounding metropolitan areas.

Our strategy is simple: First, find a hiker who knows the area and loves to hike. Second, ask that person to spend a year researching the most popular and very best trails around. And third, have that person describe each trail in terms of difficulty, scenery, condition, elevation change, and other categories of information that are important to hikers. "Pretend you've just completed a hike and met up with other hikers at the trailhead," we told each author. "Imagine their questions, and be clear in your answers."

An experienced hiker and writer, Greg Witt has selected 60 of the best hikes in and around the Salt Lake City metropolitan area. From the wilderness lakes and rocky peaks of the Wasatch Range and the Uinta Mountains to a suburban stroll along the Jordan River Parkway, Witt provides hikers (and walkers) with a great variety of outings—and all within roughly 60 miles of Salt Lake City.

You'll get more out of this book if you take a moment to read the Introduction, which explains how to read the trail listings. The "Topographic Maps" section will help you understand how useful topos are on a hike, and will also tell you where to get them. And though this is a where-to rather than a how-to guide, readers who haven't hiked extensively will find the Introduction of particular value.

As much for the opportunity to free the spirit as well as to free the body, let these hikes elevate you above the urban hurry.

All the best,
The Editors at Menasha Ridge Press

PREFACE

Alaska is our biggest, buggiest, boggiest state. Texas remains our largest unfrozen state. But mountainous Utah, if ironed out flat, would take up more space on a map than either.

—Edward Abbey

WITH MOUNTAINS ON EVERY SIDE, the Salt Lake Valley offers a greater variety of dramatic and awe-inspiring day hikes than any major metropolitan area in the United States. Nestled below the western flank of the Rockies, Salt Lake City provides ready access to a stunning array of alpine lakes, snow-draped mountain peaks, fragrant evergreen forests, deep canyon waterfalls, granite towers, and flowered cirques.

Within 60 miles of Salt Lake City there are thousands of square miles of national forest, national wilderness areas, state parks, and designated recreation areas to explore. But it takes accurate and dependable information to select the best hiking adventure for you. Within minutes of a bustling urban center, you can immerse yourself in the history of early miners, the Pony Express, the Donner Party, or Mormon pioneers. With a little planning you can summit one of a dozen 11,000-foot peaks sprinkled throughout the region. You can find solitude in flickering aspen groves, shaded canyons, and pristine wilderness. Whether you're lacing up boots, stepping into running shoes, or strapping on snowshoes, Salt Lake City is a premier destination for hikers.

ABOUT THE HIKES

It would have been easy to catalog 60 hikes near Salt Lake City from the hundreds of hiking trails in the area. But the ultimate challenge in writing *60 Hikes* was to pinpoint the

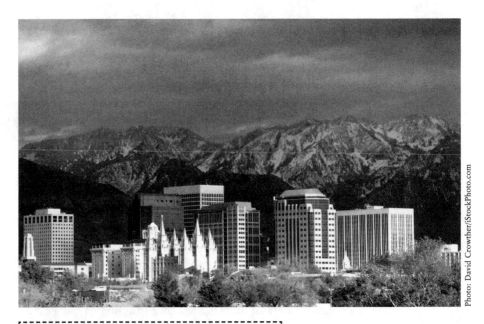

Photo: David Crowther/iStockPhoto.com

The Wasatch Mountains loom over the Salt Lake City skyline.

absolute best of those hikes—the most enjoyable, inspiring, intriguing, and accessible hikes. You'll quickly discover that every hike has a "wow factor": a memorable destination, a glistening lake, a mesmerizing stream, a breathtaking view, or a soothing canyon.

The 60 hikes that made the list had to captivate the attention of young hikers and challenge the endurance of seasoned ones. The hikes needed to reflect the diversity of the mountain, valley, and canyon terrain in the area. With rising fuel costs, I wanted to reveal hikes that were nearby and easily accessible to the 1.7 million people who live within 60 miles of Salt Lake City.

Faced with the challenge of selecting the best 60 hikes in the Salt Lake area, I assembled a powerful and compelling list in less than an hour. But the book really demanded a more rigorous process. So I distributed my best-hikes list to dozens of area hikers, rangers, scoutmasters, youth leaders, mountain bikers, rock climbers, dog walkers, trails advocates, and city recreation officials. I sought their suggestions on which hikes to include, asking them to advise which route offered the best trailhead access and best overall experience. Their input was exciting to receive and proved invaluable. Surprisingly, there was a high level of consensus on which hikes to include; in fact, the 60 hikes included here are about 90% consistent with my original list.

In order to present the most accurate information possible, I rehiked each trail to take distance measurements, determine GPS coordinates, measure elevations, and clarify trail markings. The goal was simple: create a trustworthy, authoritative trail guide that would provide years of valuable hiking pleasure.

When *60 Hikes* was first published in 2008, it instantly became the best-selling hiking guide in Utah and the essential trail guide for thousands of hikers in the Wasatch. For that I am grateful, and it's been especially enjoyable to be on the trail and run into hikers who have a well-used, dog-eared copy of *60 Hikes* in their pack.

The big challenge came with the opportunity to publish this second edition. Sure, there were some updates to include—new trailhead amenities, increased entrance fees, new access roads. But dare I take out one of my favorite hikes? And if so, which new hikes are worthy of inclusion in this second edition?

For those of you who are familiar with *60 Hikes,* as you put this second edition to the test, I think you'll be pleased with the new additions. If you're picking this book up for the first time, rest assured that you're heading to some of the most beautiful and magical places in the West. Most of all, I have loved the challenge of selecting these hikes and providing every detail to make your adventure memorable.

Just 60 hikes? Hardly. At last count it was closer to 120 hikes organized into 60 profiles. Most of the 60 hikes—indeed, most Wasatch trails—are interconnected. Each hike profile describes a particular route but also allows for options, extensions, and spur trails. In addition, the Nearby Activities mentioned at the end of most trail descriptions often reveal short hikes leading to hidden waterfalls, short interpretive trails, or points of historic or geologic interest. Most of these activities consist of walks that are less than 1 mile round-trip, while the 60 hikes are 1 mile or more in length. If you're a novice hiker and want to build your speed and stamina, you may want to start with some of the Nearby Activities.

These 60 hikes appeal to a wide variety of skill levels and interests. Of the featured hikes, about 31% are considered easy, 47% are moderate, and 22% are hard. They range in distance from 1 mile on Buffalo Peak to 16 miles on Ben Lomond. Elevation gain ranges from −58 feet on the Jordan River Parkway to 5,460 feet on Lone Peak. All the hikes are normally done as day hikes, although many can also be enjoyed as an overnight backpacking trip. You'll find that *60 Hikes* has something for everybody.

REGIONS

Hikes are organized by area in relation to Salt Lake City—north, central, south, east, and west. Conveniently, those areas also match county lines, since most of the county boundaries are defined by mountain ridges. Most of the 60 hikes are in the Wasatch Mountains, which run north and south, with the vast majority of the area's population living on the slopes and valleys to the west of the range. Within each county, hikes are organized from north to south. Here's a quick overview of each region:

NORTH (Weber County) The hikes in Weber County are easily accessed from Ogden, about 35 miles north of Salt Lake City. Ogden's historical roots as a junction on the transcontinental railroad have been overshadowed in recent years by its

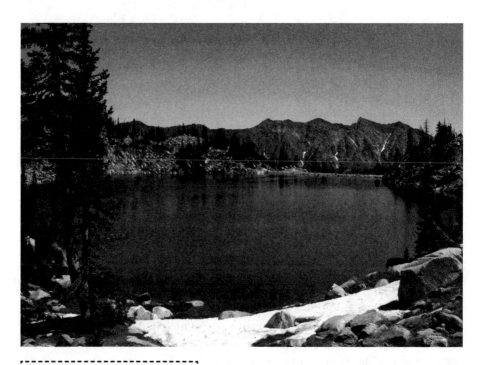

White Pine Lake (see Hike 37, page 165)

emergence as a center of outdoor recreation. The alpine peaks that hosted down-hill and super-G events in the 2002 Winter Olympic Games are also great hiking destinations in the summer. Favorite Weber County hikes include Ben Lomond to the north and beautiful Waterfall Canyon, which can be accessed just minutes from the city center.

NORTH (Davis County) Immediately north of Salt Lake City, Davis County is tradi-tionally known for farming communities such as Bountiful, Farmington, and Fruit Heights, which rest on the alluvial plain at the base of smaller Wasatch peaks. But it also offers some great canyon hikes, such as Farmington Canyon and Adams Canyon. Davis County has more square miles of Great Salt Lake than it has land area, and Antelope Island is the ideal place to explore the wonders of the lake on dry ground.

CENTRAL (Salt Lake County) It's fitting that more than half of the 60 hikes are right in Salt Lake County. These hikes offer easy access to glacial canyons, alpine lakes, and snow-capped peaks. You'll be amazed how close wilderness areas are to the heart of the city. Salt Lake's pioneer history unfolds along celebrated trails and the Pony Express route. In *60 Hikes,* you'll find adventure waiting in each of the seven canyons that have shaped, nourished, powered, and built Salt Lake City since 1847. Most hikers can find enough opportunities in Big Cottonwood Canyon alone to feed their passion for a year or more. Some of the more popular hikes in the central Wasatch include Grandeur Peak, Brighton Lakes, and Doughnut Falls.

SOUTH (Utah County) To the south of Salt Lake City, the Mount Timpanogos massif watches over Utah County. Dozens of canyons flank "Timp," and waterfalls cascade down all sides. Provo Canyon and American Fork Canyon offer exceptional year-round outdoor recreation opportunities. While Timp is arguably the best hike in northern Utah, don't overlook other Utah County jewels, such as Silver Lake and Stewart Falls.

WEST (Tooele County) With so much to enjoy in the Wasatch, you can see why most locals overlook the desert to the west. But the Stansbury Mountains and the Deseret Peak Wilderness Area, with its rugged terrain and 11,031-foot centerpiece, simply can't be ignored. Views stretch across the Bonneville Salt Flats and into Nevada. It's a straight shot out Interstate 80, just 35 miles to the west.

EAST (Uintas/Summit County) The Uinta Mountains, home to Utah's highest peaks, lie directly east of Salt Lake City, beyond the Wasatch Mountains. The Mirror Lake Scenic Byway provides easy access to picturesque basins and forests of spruce and fir. You can climb 11,943-foot Bald Mountain in less than an hour or spend days on end in the alpine heaven known as Naturalist Basin.

Let *60 Hikes* be a starting point. Let it inspire your own adventure on a road less traveled. Maybe you'll discover a hidden waterfall or encounter a mysterious field of white columbine. Wasatch trails are notoriously unmarked, and maybe with enough experience you'll discover you don't need trail signs to have a great hike. If a family of moose is blocking the trail, you may find a parallel trail over the ridge. If the trailhead parking lot is full, you can often take a shorter, steeper trail to the summit from another trailhead. The possibilities are endless, and you'll have the time of your life exploring them.

See you on the trail!

RECOMMENDED HIKES

AUTHOR'S PICKS

Best Summit Hike: Mount Timpanogos (page 204)

Best Lake Hike: Brighton Lakes (page 153)

Best Waterfall: Stewart Falls (page 212)

Best Mountain Scenery: Lofty Lake Loop (page 216)

Best Paved Trail: Timpanogos Cave National Monument (page 200)

Best Wildflowers: Cecret Lake (Albion Basin) (page 161)

Best Wildlife: Frary Peak (page 49)

Toughest Climb: Lone Peak (page 181)

HIKES OF 1–3 MILES

HIKES OF 3–6 MILES

BEST WINTER HIKES

HIKES WITH HISTORY

BEST HIKES FOR CHILDREN

BEST HIKES FOR DOGS

POPULAR TRAILS

POPULAR TRAILS *(continued)*

HIKES TO HIGH SUMMITS
(more than 10,000 feet)

HIKES WITH SWEEPING VIEWS

YEAR-ROUND HIKES

BEST HIKES FOR SOLITUDE

BEST HIKES FOR WILDLIFE

BEST HIKES FOR WILDFLOWERS

BEST FOR REGULAR WORKOUTS

SCENIC HIKES

SCENIC HIKES *(continued)*

BEST TRAILS FOR RUNNERS

The Uinta ground squirrel spends about eight months of the year in hibernation.

INTRODUCTION

Welcome to *60 Hikes within 60 Miles: Salt Lake City*. If you're new to hiking or even if you're a seasoned trailsmith, take a few minutes to read the following introduction. We explain how this book is organized and how to use it.

HOW TO USE THIS GUIDEBOOK

THE OVERVIEW MAP AND OVERVIEW-MAP KEY

Use the overview map on the inside front cover to assess the exact locations of each hike's primary trailhead. Each hike's number is listed on the overview map; on the map key facing the overview map, on the first page of the book; and in the table of contents. As you flip through the book, a hike's full profile is easy to locate by watching for the hike number at the top of most right-hand pages.

REGIONAL MAPS

The book is divided into regions, and prefacing each regional section is an overview map. The regional maps provide more detail than the overview map, bringing you closer to the hike.

TRAIL MAPS

Each hike contains a detailed map that shows the trailhead, the route, significant features, facilities, and topographic landmarks such as creeks, overlooks, and peaks. The author gathered map data by carrying a Garmin eTrex Legend GPS unit while hiking. This data was downloaded into DeLorme's Topo USA digital-mapping program and processed by expert cartographers to produce the highly accurate maps in this book. Each trailhead's GPS coordinates are included with each profile (see discussion following).

In addition to using a GPS, the author measured most trails with a measuring wheel to provide accurate distance measurements. One benefit of a measuring wheel it that it achieves greater accuracy than a GPS on steep trails with short switchbacks or in deep canyons where a satellite signal is not always obtainable.

LEGEND

A legend that explains the symbols found on trail maps appears on the inside back cover.

ELEVATION PROFILES

Each hike contains a detailed elevation profile that corresponds directly to the trail map. The elevation profile provides a quick look at the trail from the side, enabling you to visualize how the trail rises and falls. Key points along the way are labeled. Note the number of feet between each tick mark on the vertical axis (the height scale). To avoid making flat hikes look steep and steep hikes appear flat, height scales are used throughout the book to accurately depict each hike's climbing difficulty.

GPS TRAILHEAD COORDINATES

Readers can easily access all trailheads in this book by using the directions given, the overview map, and the trail map, which shows at least one major road leading into the area. But for those who enjoy using the latest GPS technology to navigate, the necessary data has been provided.

The GPS coordinates for each trailhead are presented in latitude–longitude format. These numbers tell you where you are by locating a point east or west of the prime meridian, which passes through Greenwich, England (longitude), and north or south of the equator (longitude).

For readers who own a GPS unit, whether handheld or in a vehicle, the latitude–longitude coordinates (on the first page of each hike profile) may be entered into the unit. Just make sure yours is set to navigate using the WGS84 datum. Now you can navigate directly to the trailhead.

Trailheads that begin in parking areas can be reached by car, but other hikes still require a short walk to reach the trailhead from a parking area. In those cases, a handheld GPS unit is necessary to continue the navigation process.

In this book, latitude–longitude coordinates are expressed in degrees and decimal minutes. For example, the coordinates for Hike 1, Ben Lomond (page 16), are as follows: N41° 19.236´; W111° 53.933´. To convert GPS coordinates given in degrees, minutes, and seconds to the format shown above, divide the seconds by 60. For more on GPS technology, visit **usgs.gov.**

HIKE PROFILES

Each hike contains seven key items: an In Brief description of the trail, a Key At-a-Glance Information box, directions to the trail, trailhead coordinates, a trail map, an elevation profile, and a trail description; nearly all hikes also include notes on nearby activities. Combined, the maps and information provide a clear method to assess each trail from the comfort of your favorite reading chair.

IN BRIEF

A "taste of the trail." Think of this section as a snapshot focused on the historical landmarks, beautiful vistas, and other sights you might encounter on the hike.

KEY AT-A-GLANCE INFORMATION

The following information gives you a quick idea of the statistics and specifics of each hike:

LENGTH How long the trail is from start to finish (total distance traveled). There may be options to shorten or extend the hikes, but the mileage corresponds to the described hike. Use the Description as a guide to customizing the hike for your ability or time constraints.

ELEVATION GAIN The difference in feet of elevation from the lowest point on the trail to the highest point (or occasionally vice versa, in which case the elevation gain is expressed as a negative number). For most hikes in the mountains, this will be from the trailhead (lowest point) to the summit, lake, or waterfall destination.

CONFIGURATION A description of what the trail might look like from overhead. Trails can be loops, out-and-backs (trails on which one enters and leaves along the same path), point-to-points, figure-eights, or a combination of shapes.

DIFFICULTY The degree of effort an average hiker should expect on a given hike. For simplicity, the trails are rated as *easy, moderate,* or *hard.*

SCENERY A short summary of the hike's attractions and what to expect in terms of plant life, wildlife, natural wonders, and historical features.

EXPOSURE A quick check of how much sun you can expect on your shoulders during the hike.

TRAFFIC Indicates how busy the trail might be on an average day. Trail traffic, of course, varies from day to day and season to season. Weekend days typically see the most visitors.

TRAIL SURFACE Indicates whether the trail is paved, rocky, gravel, dirt, boardwalk, or a mixture of elements.

HIKING TIME How long it takes to hike the trail. A slow but steady hiker will average 2–3 miles an hour, depending on the terrain.

WATER REQUIREMENTS Indicates a reasonable amount of water to be carried by each hiker. This amount can vary based on the daytime temperature and the availability of drinking water on the trail. Nearby sources of water that can be purified are also indicated.

SEASON Identifies the best time of year to hike the trail, taking into consideration trailhead access, trail conditions, and weather. An early-spring snowmelt or an early-fall snowstorm is always a possibility and could affect these suggestions somewhat.

ACCESS A notation of any fees or permits required to access the trail or park at the trailhead.

Mill Creek Canyon is a fee area administered by the U.S. Forest Service in cooperation with Salt Lake County, requiring a charge of $3 per vehicle as you leave the canyon. If you plan to visit the canyon frequently each year, it's worth buying the $40 annual pass.

American Fork Canyon and the **Alpine Loop Scenic Backway** in Utah County are part of the federal Recreation Fee Demonstration Program and require a fee paid at the entrance stations. A one- to three-day pass is $6, a seven-day pass is $12, and an annual pass is $45. Golden Eagle, Golden Age, and Golden Access passports are honored. Cave-tour fees at **Timpanogos Cave National Monument** are $7 per adult, $5 for juniors (ages 6–15), and $3 for children (ages 3–5), and are separate from the recreation fee paid to enter the canyon.

The **Mirror Lake Scenic Byway** in the Uintas is also a Recreation Fee Demonstration area for trail and campground users. Passes may be purchased at the Kamas Ranger Station (50 E. Center St.; 435-783-4338) or at several self-service fee stations along the highway. A daily pass is $3, a weekly pass is $6, and an annual pass is $25. Golden Age and Golden Access pass-holders receive a 50% discount.

Antelope Island State Park is the home of Frary Peak (Hike 9) and many other great day hikes. The park admission fee is $9 per vehicle or $3 for walk-ins and cyclists.

Hiking trails accessed through **Red Butte Garden** (Hike 14) require a paid admission of $8 for adults and $6 for children and seniors.

MAPS Here you'll find a list of maps that show the topography of the trail, including U.S. Geological Survey (USGS) topo quads (7.5-minute series) and Trails Illustrated maps.

FACILITIES What you can expect in terms of restrooms and water at the trailhead or nearby.

DOGS You'll want to know the applicable regulations for each hike. Dogs are not permitted in some protected watershed canyons, such as Big Cottonwood and Little Cottonwood. Mill Creek Canyon requires that dogs be leashed on even-numbered days.

SPECIAL COMMENTS These may include insider information or special considerations about the trail, access, warnings, or ideas for enhancing your hiking experience.

DIRECTIONS

Used in conjunction with the overview map, the driving directions will help you locate each trailhead from nearby interstate highway exits. Once you arrive at the trailhead, park only in designated areas.

GPS TRAILHEAD COORDINATES

The trailhead coordinates can be used in addition to the driving directions if you enter the coordinates into your GPS unit before you set out. See page 2 for additional information.

DESCRIPTION

The heart of each hike. Here, the author summarizes the trail's essence and highlights any special traits the hike has to offer. The route is clearly outlined, including any landmarks, side trips, and possible alternate routes along the way. Ultimately, the Description will help you choose which hikes are best for you.

NEARBY ACTIVITIES

Look here for information on nearby activities or points of interest. These include parks, short interpretive trails, hidden waterfalls near the highway, historical sites, museums, and restaurants. (Note that not every hike has a listing.)

WEATHER

Salt Lake City experiences a wide range of temperatures and climatic conditions in its dry four-season climate. While weather is often the single most important factor in deciding when to enjoy any given hike, many of the 60 hikes can be enjoyed year-round. However, most of the hikes in this guide lie within the Wasatch and Uinta mountain ranges, and in many cases trailheads are not accessible, trails are covered with snow, and avalanche dangers are present.

Because many of the hikes in the Wasatch and the Uintas are at high elevation, you'll find that in their short season, some of them offer a great way to beat the heat on the valley floor. As a rule of thumb, the temperature decreases about 3–5° with every 1,000 feet of elevation gained.

SALT LAKE CITY TEMPERATURE AND PRECIPITATION AVERAGES						
AVERAGE TEMPERATURE				YEARS ON RECORD: 52		
	YEAR	JAN	FEB	MAR	APR	MAY	JUN
°F	52	28	34	42	50	59	69
		JUL	AUG	SEP	OCT	NOV	DEC
°F		78	76	66	53	40	30

SALT LAKE CITY TEMPERATURE AND PRECIPITATION AVERAGES						
AVERAGE HIGH TEMPERATURE				**YEARS ON RECORD: 52**		
	YEAR	JAN	FEB	MAR	APR	MAY	JUN
°F	64	37	43	52	62	72	83
		JUL	AUG	SEP	OCT	NOV	DEC
°F		92	90	80	66	50	39
AVERAGE LOW TEMPERATURE				**YEARS ON RECORD: 52**		
	YEAR	JAN	FEB	MAR	APR	MAY	JUN
°F	40	20	24	31	38	46	54
		JUL	AUG	SEP	OCT	NOV	DEC
°F		62	61	51	40	30	22
AVERAGE PRECIPITATION				**YEARS ON RECORD: 52**		
	YEAR	JAN	FEB	MAR	APR	MAY	JUN
in.	15.6	1.3	1.2	1.8	2	1.8	0.9
		JUL	AUG	SEP	OCT	NOV	DEC
in.		0.7	0.8	1.1	1.3	1.3	1.3
AVERAGE SNOWFALL				**YEARS ON RECORD: 69**		
	YEAR	JAN	FEB	MAR	APR	MAY	JUN
in.	57.9	13.5	9.4	9.4	5	0.6	—
		JUL	AUG	SEP	OCT	NOV	DEC
in.		—	—	0.1	1.3	6.6	12

WATER

How much is enough? Well, one simple physiological fact should persuade you to err on the side of excess when deciding how much water to pack: a hiker working hard in 90°F heat needs about 10 quarts of fluid per day. That's 2.5 gallons (9.5 liters)—12 large water bottles or 16 small ones. In other words, pack along one or two bottles even for short hikes.

While it's no problem to carry adequate supplies of water on these day hikes, some hikers and backpackers hit the trail prepared to purify water found along the route. This method, while less dangerous than drinking untreated water, comes with risks if not properly performed. Purifiers with ceramic filters are the safest. Many hikers pack the slightly distasteful tetraglycine–hydroperiodide tablets to debug water (sold under the names Potable Aqua, Coughlan's, and others). Aquamira chlorine dioxide drops and tablets are nearly tasteless and almost weightless; gravity filters and hydration systems with inline filters are convenient and effective as well. SteriPEN is an ultraviolet-light treatment device that weighs about 10 ounces.

If none of these methods is available, bringing the water to a boil is enough to kill the pathogens.

Probably the most common waterborne bug that hikers face is giardia, which may not hit until one to four weeks after ingestion. It will have you living in the bathroom, passing noxious rotten-egg gas, vomiting, and shivering with chills. Other parasites to worry about include E. coli and cryptosporidium, both of which are harder to kill than giardia.

For most people, the pleasures of hiking make carrying water a relatively minor price to pay to remain healthy. If you're tempted to drink "found water," do so only if you understand the risks involved. Better yet, hydrate prior to your hike, carry (and drink) 6 ounces of water for every mile you plan to hike, and hydrate after the hike.

GEAR
CLOTHING

For most hikes in the summer season, your choice of trail clothing can vary widely and is really more a matter of personal preference. Shorts or long pants? Long-sleeve or short-sleeve shirt? Those are probably decisions you'll make the morning of the hike without much thought. For longer, more strenuous hikes, you may want to consider synthetic moisture-wicking fabric instead of cotton, which retains moisture and can even lead to hypothermia if the temperature drops quickly. It's a good idea to pack a lightweight fleece or an extra outer layer for higher elevations or in case of a surprise drop in temperature.

When it comes to footwear, comfort and personal preference should be your guides. Since these are all day hikes and don't require a heavy pack, you may find that a lightweight trail shoe is your best bet. Athletic shoes may be sufficient for paved trails and short hikes of less than 3 miles. For longer hikes and those involving steep, rocky terrain, you'll want to consider a hiking shoe with a thick, firm, supportive sole.

THE TEN ESSENTIALS

One of the first rules of hiking is to be prepared for anything. The simplest way to be prepared is to carry the ten essentials. In addition to carrying the items listed below and on the next page, you need to know how to use them, especially navigation items. Always consider worst-case scenarios such as getting lost, hiking back in the dark, broken gear (for example, a broken hip strap on your pack or a water filter that gets plugged), twisting an ankle, or a brutal thunderstorm. The listed items don't cost a lot of money, don't take up much room in a pack, and don't weigh much, but they might just save your life.

COMPASS: A high-quality model

EXTRA CLOTHES: Rain protection, warm layers, gloves, socks, warm hat

EXTRA FOOD: You should always have food in your pack when you've finished hiking

FIRE: Windproof matches or lighter and fire starter

FIRST-AID KIT: A good-quality kit including instructions

KNIFE: A multitool device with pliers is best

LIGHT: Flashlight or headlamp with extra bulbs and batteries

MAP: Preferably a topo map and a trail map with a route description

SUN PROTECTION: Sunglasses, lip balm, sunscreen, sun hat

WATER: Durable bottles and water treatment, like iodine or a filter

FIRST-AID KIT

A typical first-aid kit may contain more items than you think necessary. The following items are just the basics. Prepackaged kits in waterproof bags are available (Atwater Carey and Adventure Medical Kits are a couple of brands). Even though quite a few items are listed here, they pack down into a small space:

Ace bandages or Spenco joint wraps

Adhesive bandages

Antibiotic ointment (Neosporin or the generic equivalent)

Aspirin or acetaminophen

Benadryl or the generic equivalent, diphenhydramine (in case of allergic reactions)

Butterfly-closure bandages

Epinephrine in a prefilled syringe (for people known to have severe allergic reactions to such things as bee stings)

Gauze (one roll and a half-dozen 4 by 4–inch compress pads)

Hydrogen peroxide or iodine

Insect repellent

Matches or pocket lighter

Moleskin/Spenco 2nd Skin

Sunscreen

Whistle (it's more effective in signaling rescuers than your voice)

HIKING WITH CHILDREN

No one is too young for a hike in the outdoors. Be mindful, though. Flat, short, and shaded trails are best with an infant. Toddlers who haven't quite mastered walking can still tag along, riding on an adult's back in a child carrier. Use common sense to judge a child's capacity to hike a particular trail, and be ready for the child to tire quickly and need to be carried.

When packing for the hike, remember the child's needs as well as your own. Make sure children are adequately clothed for the weather, have proper shoes, and are protected from the sun with sunscreen. Kids dehydrate quickly, so make sure you have plenty of fluids for everyone. Hikes suitable for children are noted on page xix.

GENERAL SAFETY

To some potential hikers, mountain peaks, canyons, and wilderness areas seem perilous. No doubt, potentially dangerous situations can occur outdoors, but if you use sound judgment and prepare yourself before hitting the trail, you'll be much safer in the woods or mountains than in most urban areas of the country. It's better to look at a backcountry hike as a fascinating chance to discover the unknown rather than a setting for potential disaster. These tips will help make your trip safer and easier.

- **ALWAYS CARRY FOOD AND WATER,** whether you plan to go overnight or not. Food will give you energy, help keep you warm, and sustain you in an emergency situation until help arrives. You never know if you'll have a stream nearby when you become thirsty. Bring potable water, or treat water before drinking it from a stream or other source.

- **STAY ON DESIGNATED TRAILS.** Most hikers get lost when they leave the path. Even on the most clearly marked trails, you usually reach a point where you have to stop and consider the direction in which to head. If you become disoriented, don't panic. As soon as you think you may be off-track, stop, assess your current direction, and then retrace your steps back to the point where you went awry. Using a map, compass, and this book—and keeping in mind what you've passed thus far—reorient yourself, and trust your judgment about which way to continue. If you become absolutely unsure of how to continue, return to your vehicle the way you came in. Should you become completely lost and have no idea how to return to the trailhead, remaining in place along the trail and waiting for help is most often the best option for adults and always the best option for children.

- **BE ESPECIALLY CAREFUL WHEN CROSSING STREAMS.** Whether you're fording the stream or crossing on a log, make every step count. If you're not sure you can maintain your balance on a foot log, ford the stream instead. When fording a stream, use a trekking pole or stout stick for balance and face upstream as you cross. If a stream seems too deep to ford, turn back. Whatever is on the other side is not worth risking your life.

- **BE CAREFUL AT OVERLOOKS.** While these areas may provide spectacular views, they are potentially hazardous. Stay back from the edge of outcrops, and be absolutely sure of your footing.

- **STANDING DEAD TREES AND STORM-DAMAGED LIVING TREES POSE A HAZARD** to hikers and tent campers. These trees may have loose or broken limbs that could fall at any time. When choosing a spot to rest or camp, look up.

- **KNOW THE SYMPTOMS OF HEAT EXHAUSTION.** Excessive sweating, faintness or dizziness, clammy skin, vomiting, and paleness are all common symptoms. If symptoms arise, remove extra clothing, move to the shade, and drink plenty of water.

- **LIKEWISE, KNOW THE SYMPTOMS OF HYPOTHERMIA.** Shivering and forgetfulness are the two most common indicators of this insidious killer. Hypothermia can occur at any elevation, even in the summer, especially when the hiker is wearing lightweight cotton clothing. Get the victim shelter, hot liquids, and dry clothes or a dry sleeping bag.

- **BRING YOUR BRAIN.** A cool, calculating mind is the single most important piece of equipment you'll ever need on the trail. Think before you act. Watch your step. Plan ahead. Avoiding accidents before they happen is the best recipe for a rewarding and relaxing hike.

- **ASK QUESTIONS.** Forest and park employees are there to help. It's a lot easier to gain advice beforehand and avoid a mishap away from civilization, where it's too late to amend an error. Use your head out there, and treat the place as if it were your own backyard.

NATURAL HAZARDS

The two most deadly natural hazards in Utah are lightning and avalanche. The best way, and really the only way, to protect yourself from these hazards is to avoid the areas and conditions where they are most likely to occur. Although many of the chapters in this book identify areas that are particularly avalanche- or lightning-prone, you should always observe posted warnings, check weather advisories, watch local conditions, and use a healthy dose of common sense before venturing into the backcountry.

LIGHTNING

Most summer hikes in the Wasatch take place in favorable weather under cloud-free skies; still, afternoon thunderstorms can always roll in. If you see a storm approaching, or if you can see lightning or hear thunder, the risk is already present. Louder or more frequent thunder means electrical activity is approaching, increasing the risk of lightning injury or death. If the time delay between seeing the lightning and hearing the thunder is less than 30 seconds, you're in danger.

No place is absolutely safe from the threat of lightning, but some places are safer than others. Seek covered shelter as quickly as possible. Avoid being on or near ridgelines, mountain peaks, exposed slopes, open fields, isolated trees, communications towers, ski-lift supports, metal fences, or water.

AVALANCHE

While climbers, backcountry skiers, and snowmobilers are the most likely avalanche victims in Utah, snowshoers and recreational hikers can also be at risk. Avalanches can occur on any slope given the right snow conditions. Hikers should observe avalanche warnings and check local avalanche advisory services before entering the backcountry in wintertime. Avalanches are most likely to occur in areas where they've occurred in the past, particularly near steep, barren slopes and in the presence of avalanche-scarred terrain.

ANIMAL HAZARDS

MOUNTAIN LIONS

As more people get into the outdoors and encroach upon wildlife habitat, human encounters with mountain lions (a.k.a. cougars or pumas) are bound to increase. Although sightings of this elusive species are extremely rare, mountain lions live throughout the Wasatch and Uinta mountains. These animals are unlikely to attack an adult human, but in the event of an encounter, make yourself as big and loud as you can. Try growling, baring your teeth, raising your arms, or fanning out your jacket. Act threatening, but give the mountain lion an escape path. Never crouch down or turn your back on the animal, and don't approach it. Don't run away—that can trigger the cat's chasing instincts. Make noise, yell, and throw rocks or anything you can grab without bending over. Lastly, if there are young children nearby, keep them close and even lift them on your shoulders if you can.

If you're attacked, try to remain standing, as mountain lions will try to bite the neck or head. Always try to fight back.

BEARS

Black bears, the only bear species found in Utah, are relatively common in mountain forests. Although they are more likely to be found near campgrounds in search of food, they can also be seen on backcountry trails. Generally, they avoid contact with people and will usually run away.

Bears want your food, so take every precaution to keep it under your control. Do not leave food out and unattended. If a bear is already eating your food or shredding your pack in search of snacks, let him have it. Perhaps you can walk away with just a great story.

If you do encounter a black bear on the trail, don't run. Avoid cornering the animal or coming between a cub and its mother. Back away slowly, and make loud noises to scare it away. Make eye contact, but don't stare. Pick up small children to keep them from running. If a bear approaches, make yourself appear larger by spreading your arms or holding your jacket open. Make as much threatening noise as you can by yelling or banging gear together. If a bear is after you and not your food, throw rocks or sticks and make every attempt to fight back.

MOOSE

Sightings of moose in Wasatch meadows and canyon drainages are common and generally quite enjoyable. It's a good time to pull out your camera. While moose aren't aggressive, they may charge when they perceive a threat. Do not approach or engage the moose.

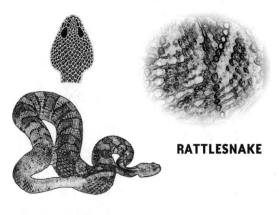

RATTLESNAKE

SNAKES

Rattlesnakes are most commonly found on dry, south-facing foot-hill slopes, where they enjoy sunning themselves on the trail. It's not uncommon to nearly step on the snake before you see it. Rat-tlesnakes aren't aggressive and will usually slither off if given a chance. If the snake won't move out of your way as you approach, you can usually get it to move by tossing a rock or stick in its direction.

Rattlesnakes will not attack, but they will defend themselves if disturbed or cornered. They will usually warn you with the buzz of their rattle. Be careful when you step over logs or boulders. Don't place your foot in a spot you can't see. Watch where you place your hands when scrambling. Snakebites most often occur when you inadvertently touch the snake.

MOSQUITOES

Mosquitoes are not a significant problem for hikers on sunlit Wasatch mountain trails, but cases of West Nile virus have been reported in Utah. Because West Nile is spread primarily by the bite of an infected mosquito, you should consider using a mosquito repellent with DEET or Picaridin, especially from dusk to dawn, when mosquitoes are most active.

TOPOGRAPHIC MAPS

The maps in this book have been produced with great care and, used with the hiking directions, will direct you to the trail and help you stay on-course. However, you will find superior detail and valuable information in the USGS's 7.5-minute series topo-graphic maps. One well-known free topo service on the Web is **Microsoft Research Maps (msrmaps.com)**, which also offers satellite imagery. Online services such as **Trails .com** charge annual fees for additional features such as shaded relief, which makes the topography stand out more. If you expect to print out many topo maps each year, it might be worth paying for such extras. The downside to USGS topos is that most are outdated, having been created 20–30 years ago. But they still provide excellent topographic detail.

Digital programs such as DeLorme's Topo North America enable you to review topo maps on your computer. Data gathered while hiking with a GPS unit can be downloaded into the software, letting you plot your own hikes. Of course, **Google Earth (earth.google.com)** does away with topo maps and their inaccuracies, replacing them with satellite imagery and its inaccuracies. Regardless, what one lacks the other augments. Google Earth is an excellent tool whether or not you have difficulty with topos.

If you're new to hiking, you might be wondering, "What's a topographic map?" In short, a topo indicates not only linear distance but elevation as well, using contour lines. These lines spread across the map like dozens of intricate spiderwebs. Each line represents a particular elevation, and at the base of each topo a contour's interval designation is given. If the contour interval is 20 feet, then the distance between each contour line is 20 feet. Follow five contour lines up on the same map, and the elevation has increased by 100 feet.

Let's assume that the 7.5-minute-series topo reads "contour interval 40 feet," that the short trail we'll be hiking is 2 inches in length on the map, and that it crosses five contour lines from beginning to end. What do we know? Well, because the linear scale of this series is 2,000 feet to the inch (roughly 2.75 inches representing 1 mile), we know that our trail is about three-fourths of a mile long (2 inches equals 4,000 feet). But we also know we'll be climbing or descending 200 vertical feet (five contour lines are 40 feet each) over that distance. And the elevation designations written on occasional contour lines will tell us if we're heading up or down.

In addition to the outdoor shops listed in Appendix A, you'll find topos at major universities and some public libraries. If you want your own and can't find them locally, visit **nationalmap.gov** or **store.usgs.gov**.

TRAIL ETIQUETTE

Whether you're on a city, county, state, or national-park trail, always remember that great care and resources (from nature as well as from your tax dollars) have gone into creating these trails. Treat the trail, wildlife, and fellow hikers with respect.

- **Hike on open trails only. Respect trail and road closures (ask if you're not sure), avoid possible trespassing on private land, and obtain all permits and authorization as required. Also, leave gates as you found them or as marked.**

- **Leave only footprints. Be sensitive to the ground beneath you. This also means staying on the existing trail and not blazing any new trails. Pack out what you pack in. No one likes to see the trash someone else has left behind.**

- **Never spook animals. An unannounced approach, a sudden movement, or a loud noise can startle them. A surprised animal can be dangerous to you, others, and itself. Give animals plenty of space.**

- **Plan ahead. Know your equipment, your ability, and the area in which you are hiking—and prepare accordingly. Be self-sufficient at all times; carry necessary supplies for changes in weather or other conditions. A well-executed trip is a satisfaction to you and to others.**

- **Be courteous to other hikers, bikers, equestrians, and others you encounter on the trails. Hikers and bikers should yield to equestrians, bikers should yield to hikers, and, whenever safe, everyone should yield to uphill hikers, bikers, or equestrians.**

   When you encounter equestrians, it's very helpful to move off-trail to the downhill side and greet the rider. This helps the horse understand that you aren't a threat.

North: Weber County (Hikes 1–5)

North Ogden

N. Ogden Canyon Road

UINTA-WASATCH-CACHE NATIONAL FOREST

Lewis Peak

N. Fork Ogden River

Pineview Reservoir

Ogden River

Snowbasin Road

MOUNT OGDEN PARK

Mount Ogden

0 1 2 3 miles
0 1 2 3 kilometers

NORTH
(WEBER COUNTY)

1   BEN LOMOND

KEY AT-A-GLANCE INFORMATION

LENGTH: 16 miles round-trip

ELEVATION GAIN: 3,532'

ELEVATION AT TRAILHEAD: 6,180'

CONFIGURATION: Out-and-back

DIFFICULTY: Hard

SCENERY: Views of Ogden Valley and Great Salt Lake along the ridgeline, with panoramic views from the summit

EXPOSURE: Partially shaded to saddle, unshaded from saddle to summit

TRAFFIC: Light

TRAIL SURFACE: Dirt with rock near summit

HIKING TIME: 8–9 hours

WATER REQUIREMENTS: 2–3 liters; no water on or near trail

SEASON: Late spring–early fall

ACCESS: No fees or permits

MAPS: USGS North Ogden

FACILITIES: Restrooms at trailhead but no water

DOGS: On leash

SPECIAL COMMENTS: This is a long, dry trail. Come prepared with adequate water, food, and sun protection.

GPS TRAILHEAD COORDINATES

N41° 19.236´ W111° 53.933´

IN BRIEF

Ben Lomond has the longest, most gentle gradient of any summit trail in the Wasatch. Along the way you're treated to continuous and commanding views in all directions, with a diverse range of vegetation and wildlife.

DESCRIPTION

The best known of the northern Wasatch peaks dominates the skyline over North Ogden. An early pioneer named the peak Ben Lomond because it reminded her of the mountain of the same name in her native Scotland. Years later, W. W. Hodkinson, who lived in Ogden as a young man, drew inspiration from Ben Lomond when he founded Paramount Pictures in 1914. Hodkinson designed the familiar logo of a towering snowcapped peak.

While several routes lead to the Ben Lomond summit, the North Skyline Trail (which is also a section of the Great Western Trail) offers a particularly scenic and varied ascent. Although the North Skyline Trail is a bit longer than the other trails that ascend from the east, it is well traveled, it's reliable, and it offers a wider variety of views along the route, to both the east and west.

From the North Ogden Divide trailhead, cross North Ogden Canyon Road and start making your way up a series of 12 sweeping

----

Directions

Take I-15 north from Salt Lake City to 12th Street in Ogden (Exit 344). Go east 2.3 miles on 12th Street to Washington Boulevard. Turn left on Washington Boulevard (US 89) and go north 5.1 miles to 31st Street. Turn right on 31st Street and continue 4.1 miles to the North Ogden Divide trailhead parking area, on the right.

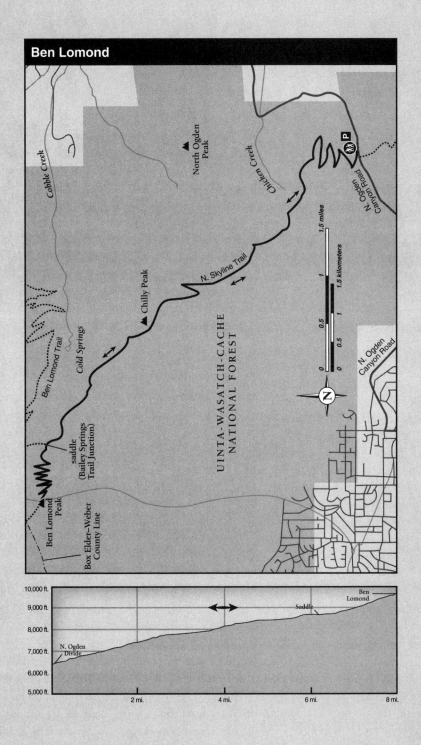

Ben Lomond

North Ogden Peak

Cobble Creek

Chicken Creek

N. Ogden Canyon Road

N. Skyline Trail

Chilly Peak

Ben Lomond Trail

Cold Springs

UINTA-WASATCH-CACHE NATIONAL FOREST

N. Ogden Canyon Road

saddle (Bailey Springs Trail Junction)

Ben Lomond Peak

Box Elder–Weber County Line

1.5 miles
1.5 kilometers
1
1
0.5
0.5
0

10,000 ft.
9,000 ft.
8,000 ft.
7,000 ft.
6,000 ft.
5,000 ft.

Ben Lomond
Saddle
N. Ogden Divide

2 mi.   4 mi.   6 mi.   8 mi.

Ben Lomond's summit from the western ridge trail

switchbacks that lead up the north side of the mountain over the course of 2.5 miles. As you ascend through a dense cover of Gambel oak, maple, and curly-leaf mountain mahogany, watch out for rattlesnakes that enjoy sunning themselves on the south-facing trail.

Beyond the switchbacks, you'll enter a long traverse along the ridge's eastern slope where aspens, bent by heavy snow accumulation, continually lean to the east. This section of trail leads through deer brush (a mountain shrub found throughout the West) and offers generous views of Ogden Valley to the east. Soon the trail enters mature stands of fir and spruce, which provide some shade. Along this ridge you'll have views stretching from Morgan County in the south to 9,979-foot Naomi Peak near the Idaho border in the north.

At 4.2 miles from the trailhead and an elevation of 8,240 feet, the trail crosses to the west side of the ridge and yields your first view of the Ben Lomond summit to the northwest. The trail continues straight ahead (northwest) for another 2.3 miles, gaining just over 500 feet in elevation on slopes blanketed with deer brush and dotted with limber pine.

Arriving at the Bailey Springs Trail junction, commonly known as the saddle, you'll find a large wooden sign with a map showing other trails on the mountain, trail distances, and various points of interest. From this saddle the trail continues to the northwest with the summit in clear view. You're most likely to see mountain goats on rocky slopes at these higher elevations. Above the windswept saddle, krummholz limber pine and subalpine fir dot the grassy slopes, along with lupine.

In the remaining 1.5 miles and 900 vertical feet to the summit, the trail steepens somewhat, but never enough to become grueling. The final summit approach is accomplished with a well-crafted chain of 28 short switchbacks through outcrops of quartzite, slate, and schist. The well-established trail will take you directly to the summit without your ever having to scramble, boulder-hop, or bushwhack.

At the 9,712-foot summit, the views stretch out in all directions, with Willard Bay and the Great Salt Lake being the dominant features to the west. Directly to your north is Willard Peak, which at 9,764 feet is the highest point in Weber County and a tad higher than Ben Lomond—a fact that comes as a surprise to many hikers. A straightforward traverse along a trail to the north can lead you on to Willard Peak, adding several hours to an already-long day.

Ben Lomond is a classic northern Utah climb: thoroughly enjoyable, yet very different from the southern Wasatch peaks with their high-elevation trailheads and canyon approaches. On the long descent, come prepared with enough water to keep you hydrated. The afternoon sun beats down on the dry, unshaded, south-facing switchbacks that return you to the trailhead.

NEARBY ACTIVITIES

The **Ogden Nature Center** is a 152-acre wildlife sanctuary and education center at 966 W. 12th St. in Ogden. The land is home to mule deer, pheasants, fox, and migrating birds. More than 1.5 miles of walking trails make the sanctuary and ponds accessible. The visitor center features hands-on exhibits, an observation beehive, and The Nest gift shop, with nature-related gifts for all ages. For events and information, call 801-621-7595 or visit **ogdennaturecenter.org**.

2 OGDEN RIVER PARKWAY

KEY AT-A-GLANCE INFORMATION

LENGTH: 3.4 miles one-way (recommended portion, 2 miles one-way)

ELEVATION GAIN: −132' (recommended portion, −73')

ELEVATION AT TRAILHEAD: 4,432'

CONFIGURATION: One-way or out-and-back

DIFFICULTY: Easy

SCENERY: River, parks, and mountain views

EXPOSURE: Mostly shaded

TRAFFIC: Moderate

TRAIL SURFACE: Asphalt

HIKING TIME: 1–2 hours

WATER REQUIREMENTS: 0.5 liter

SEASON: Year-round

ACCESS: 1 hour before sunrise–1 hour after sunset; no fees or permits

MAPS: USGS Ogden

FACILITIES: Restrooms, water, and other services at trailhead and at various parks along the way

DOGS: On leash

SPECIAL COMMENTS: Skateboarding, horses, and motorized vehicles are prohibited on the parkway. Bicycle speed limit is 10 mph.

GPS TRAILHEAD COORDINATES

N41° 14.202´ W111° 55.773´

IN BRIEF

The Ogden River emerges from Ogden Canyon, cuts through Ogden, and flows west toward the Great Salt Lake. Along the way, the Ogden River Parkway connects many of Ogden's most popular parks and recreational venues. The parkway currently extends 3.4 miles, but the most scenic and enjoyable section is the first 1.4 miles, from the mouth of Ogden Canyon to the Ogden Botanical Gardens.

DESCRIPTION

As it emerges from the mouth of Ogden Canyon, the Ogden River still thinks it's a mountain stream. It tumbles and careens off large boulders, its banks lined with the quaking aspens and bigtooth maples common to mountain tributaries. But as it enters the city limits, the river becomes more urban. Its pace slows, and the boulders give way to dirt banks. Towering cottonwoods—characteristic of desert streams—replace the aspens and maples. The Ogden River Parkway parallels the river and captures the transformation.

The best place to start a walk along the parkway is at the canyon-mouth trailhead,

----

Directions ⟶

Take I-15 north from Salt Lake City to 21st Street/UT 401 (Exit 343) in Ogden. Curve right and continue east 3.2 miles to Harrison Boulevard (UT 203). Turn left on Harrison Boulevard and continue north 0.8 mile to Canyon Road (UT 39). Turn right on Canyon Road and continue east 1 mile toward the mouth of Ogden Canyon. At Valley Drive (1700 South) turn right, then enter the Rainbow Gardens parking lot, to the left. The trailhead is across the street, at the corner of Valley Drive and Park Boulevard (1900 East).

Ogden River Parkway

UINTA-WASATCH-CACHE
NATIONAL FOREST

Mount Ogden from Big Dee Sports Park

across the street from Rainbow Gardens, an Ogden resort and recreation area since 1895. Because there's no parking at the trailhead, you may want to park your car in the large parking lot at Rainbow Gardens, stop by the gift shop for water and trail snacks, and use the restrooms.

While it is officially designated as a multiuse trail, the Ogden River Parkway does not allow skateboards or horses. In addition, bicycles have a 10-mph speed limit, which encourages the more avid and aggressive cyclists to go elsewhere.

For the first 0.3 mile, the trail is pinned between the river on the right and Park Boulevard on the left. Then the street diverges from the trail while the path continues to hug the river. The trail stays close to the river throughout, providing frequent opportunities to access the water.

The trail's upper portion maintains a playful, parklike, recreational feel. For the first 2.5 miles, until the parkway crosses Washington Boulevard (US 89), the trail and river link a continuous series of parks, playgrounds, sports fields, George S. Eccles Dinosaur Park, a skateboard park, a rodeo arena, El Monte Golf Course, and Ogden Botanical Gardens.

Park benches every 100 feet or so provide plenty of opportunities to sit and enjoy the river or take a break for a picnic. The string of parks and recreation areas also offers easy access to drinking water and restrooms along the asphalt trail.

At 1 mile from the trailhead, the trail forks. Stay to the right, on the river side. At 1.4 miles, you'll arrive at the beautiful Ogden Botanical Gardens. Here you'll have access to water, a public phone, restrooms, and a covered picnic area,

Ogden River

making it an ideal spot to stop for a rest, enjoy the gardens, have a picnic, or start back to the trailhead.

If you decide to continue beyond the botanical gardens, the river slows and the parkway takes on an older, more run-down feeling. It passes junkyards, brick-yards, old motels, and public storage units. Although the trail remains close to the river, it's often bound by a fence on both sides. The trail finally crosses over a large railroad yard at the 20th Street Bridge, continues around the 21st Street Pond, and then joins the Weber River Parkway at the confluence of the Ogden and Weber rivers in a scenic, shaded setting. From the trailhead to the 20th Street Bridge is 3.4 miles one-way. But you'll find most of the trail's vibrancy and scenic enjoyment in the first 2 miles, making the Botanical Gardens a recommended turnaround point.

The Ogden River merges with the Weber River just east of I-15 and flows another 10 miles, flattening into a wetlands delta that empties into the Great Salt Lake. At the Ogden River Parkway trailhead, hikers can also easily connect with the Bonneville Shoreline Trail for access to some of Mount Ogden's most popular trails.

NEARBY ACTIVITIES

The **Ogden Botanical Gardens** are on the Ogden River Parkway, 1.4 miles downriver (west) from the trailhead at 1750 Monroe Blvd. An extension program of Utah State University, the gardens feature more than 11 acres of landscaped grounds and facil-ities for weddings and large group events. Open year-round; for additional informa-tion, call 801-399-8080 or visit **ogdenbotanicalgardens.blogspot.com.**

3 MOUNT OGDEN (via Snowbasin Gondola)

KEY AT-A-GLANCE INFORMATION

LENGTH: 3.1 miles round-trip

ELEVATION GAIN: 862' on foot + 2,310' by gondola

ELEVATION: 6,415' (Needles Gondola Base), 8,710' (Needles Lodge)

CONFIGURATION: Out-and-back

DIFFICULTY: Easy

SCENERY: Glacial bowl, ridgeline, and great views on all sides

EXPOSURE: No shade

TRAFFIC: Moderate

TRAIL SURFACE: Dirt, rock

HIKING TIME: 2–2.5 hours

WATER REQUIREMENTS: 1 liter

SEASON: Summer

ACCESS: Hike lies on U.S. Forest Service land accessed through Snowbasin Ski Resort. You must buy a ticket to ride the gondola to Needles Lodge; summer rates: $14 adults, $5 ages 7–17, free for children age 6 and younger.

MAPS: USGS Snowbasin, Ogden

FACILITIES: Restrooms, water, phones, equipment rentals, dining, and shopping at the base in Grizzly Center and at Earl's Lodge; restrooms, water, and phones at Needles Lodge

DOGS: Not permitted on gondola

GPS TRAILHEAD COORDINATES

Needles Gondola Base:
N41° 12.945´ W111° 51.438´
Needles Lodge:
N41° 11.617´ W111° 52.440´

IN BRIEF

You'll gain most of your elevation on the gondola ride, which tops out near a glacial cirque. From there, it's just 20 minutes to the ridgeline. A faint trail follows the ridgeline to the summit, offering sweeping views in all directions.

DESCRIPTION

As with many of Utah's ski resorts, Snowbasin has an appeal that extends far beyond ski season. Summer is a great time to play in the mountains and take advantage of a beautiful setting with available resort features. The same slopes that challenged skiers in the downhill and super-G events at the 2002 Olympic Winter Games test the skills of hikers and mountain bikers in the summer.

You can climb to Mount Ogden's summit from Beus Canyon or Malans Basin on its western slopes. You can also start at the base of the Snowbasin Resort and hike your way up slopes of Douglas-fir and white fir, although much of the route takes you along resort service roads (4 miles one-way from the resort to the summit). By riding the gondola to Needles

- -

Directions ————————→

Take I-15 north from Salt Lake City to US 89 (Exit 324) in Farmington, leading to I-84 east. Continue north 10.5 miles on US 89 to I-84. Veer right onto I-84 going east toward Morgan. Go 4.4 miles to Mountain Green/Huntsville (Exit 92). At the off-ramp, turn left to cross under I-84 and turn right onto UT 167 toward Snowbasin. Continue 1.5 miles on UT 167 as it turns left toward Huntsville. At 7 miles from the I-84 exit, turn left onto UT 226 and continue 3.3 miles to the main parking area. The Needles Gondola departs from the area in front of Grizzly Center.

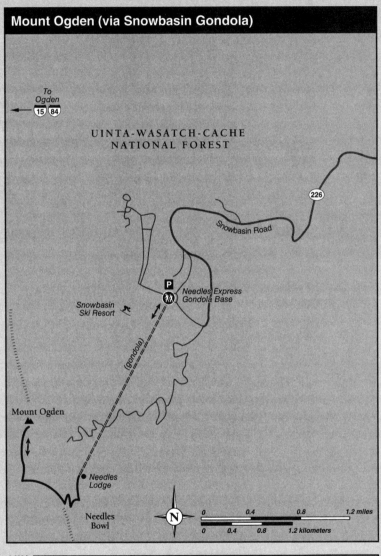

Mount Ogden (via Snowbasin Gondola)

To Ogden
15 84

UINTA-WASATCH-CACHE
NATIONAL FOREST

226

Snowbasin Road

P
Needles Express
Gondola Base

Snowbasin
Ski Resort

(gondola)

Mount Ogden

Needles
Lodge

Needles
Bowl

N

0   0.4   0.8   1.2 miles

0   0.4   0.8   1.2 kilometers

9,600 ft.   Mount
                                                                     Ogden
9,400 ft.

9,200 ft.

9,000 ft.

8,800 ft.

8,600 ft.

        0.25 mi.   0.5 mi.   0.75 mi.   1 mi.   1.25 mi.   1.5 mi.

Mount Ogden viewed from Snowbasin

Lodge at 8,710 feet, you can hike to the summit and back in a little more than 2 hours and still have time for mountain biking, an afternoon round of disc golf, or a mountain picnic. The hike to the summit from Needles Lodge is also a good choice for families or less experienced hikers who want to reach a recognizable summit on a trail that matches their experience levels. During the summer the gondola operates Friday, Saturday, and Sunday. If you hike up, you can ride down at no charge.

The gondola achieves 2,310 feet of vertical lift in about 1.7 miles. In summer, the leisurely ride takes about 18 minutes, in ski season about 15 minutes. After the gondola reaches Needles Lodge, exit the platform and turn left, following the signs that lead you to the Needles Loop Trail and the Cirque Practice Loop to the southwest. You will take the Cirque Practice Loop to the right.

At 0.2 mile from Needles Lodge on the Cirque Practice Loop, you'll see a sign pointing to the Needles Cirque Trail to the ridge. Here you depart the mountain-bike trail for a footpath. Follow this faint trail as it switchbacks up this grassy cirque to the ridge. Deer frequently graze in this cirque, and a large patch of snow often remains until midsummer.

Once at the 9,062-foot saddle, you'll enjoy views down Beus Canyon to your west, beyond Hill Air Force Base and stretching far beyond the Great Salt Lake. Mount Ogden lies along the ridgeline to the north and can be recognized by the communications towers on its summit. At this saddle, three unnamed peaks, or knolls, compose the ridgeline between you and the Mount Ogden summit.

A faint trail follows a gentle contour along the western slopes of these first two knolls. Below, you'll see the Beus Canyon Trail winding its way up the dry slopes. Along this part of the trail, you'll be hiking on slopes covered with sage and dotted with an occasional limber pine or subalpine fir. Rattlesnakes frequently bask in the sun on this section of trail, so keep your eyes wide open.

After you round the second knoll, the faint trail has all but vanished. You have two options at this point: drop to a lower visible trail to the left of the third knoll, or ascend the sage slope, crossing over the saddle on the south of the third knoll and arriving at the saddle to the south of Mount Ogden from the east. Most hikers favor crossing the saddle at this point. As you descend the eastern slope of this third knoll, you arrive at a service road and a concrete bunker that shields some propane tanks.

From here, follow the steep service road that leads to the summit. At 0.2 mile along the service road, take a marked foot trail to your right that ascends the rocky slope to capture the summit. On the 9,572-foot summit you'll be just a few feet higher than the helipad to your west. You'll have great views in all directions, with some wonderful direct views of Ben Lomond peak to the north and Pineview Reservoir to the east.

NEARBY ACTIVITIES

Snowbasin's summer activities include an 18-hole disc-golf course and 25 miles of hiking and mountain-biking trails. Special events include moonlit gondola rides and star parties, summer concerts, guided mountain-bike rides and races, outdoor learning excursions, and award-winning dining. Call 801-620-1000 or visit **snowbasin** **.com** for events and schedules.

4 MALANS PEAK (via Taylor Canyon)

KEY AT-A-GLANCE INFORMATION

LENGTH: 5 miles round-trip

ELEVATION GAIN: 2,200'

ELEVATION AT TRAILHEAD: 4,780'

CONFIGURATION: Out-and-back

DIFFICULTY: Moderate

SCENERY: Deep canyon, natural spring, exceptional views

EXPOSURE: Mostly shaded above bench

TRAFFIC: Bench trails are busy; the trail from Taylor Canyon to Malans Peak is uncrowded.

TRAIL SURFACE: Dirt, rock

HIKING TIME: 2–3 hours

WATER REQUIREMENTS: 1 liter; water from Malans Springs is safe at the source

SEASON: Year-round; negligible avalanche risk in lower Taylor Canyon

ACCESS: No fees or permits. Trailhead parking lot and gates close at dusk.

MAPS: USGS Ogden

FACILITIES: No restrooms or water at trailhead

DOGS: On leash

GPS TRAILHEAD COORDINATES

N41° 12.644´ W111° 55.917´

IN BRIEF

In just under 2.5 miles, you go from city neighborhoods to brushy bench to a deep canyon and spring-fed creek. Ascending the steep slope, you're rewarded with one of the best views in the area.

DESCRIPTION

Some might claim that Malans Peak really isn't a peak at all, just a rocky outcrop in the foothills of Mount Ogden's western slopes. But the commanding views and the wooded trail leading up the northern slope make this a satisfying hike and a worthwhile destination. You can most easily reach Malans Peak from Taylor Canyon, the large canyon on the north side of Mount Ogden, starting at the east end of 27th Street in Ogden.

The peak was named for Bartholomew "Tim" Malan, a prominent Ogdenite. In 1892, Malan and his family carved a road up Taylor Canyon, where they built Malan Heights Hotel in the basin between Malans Peak and Mount Ogden. Malan hauled visitors to the hotel in a wagon with a trailing "poke stick" to keep it from rolling backward. Guests received

----

Directions

Take I-15 north from Salt Lake City to 31st Street in Ogden (Exit 341A). Go east 1.1 miles on 31st Street to Washington Boulevard (US 89) and turn left. Go north 0.1 mile to 30th Street and turn right. Continue east 1.3 miles on 30th Street to Tyler Avenue (1300 East) and turn left. Go north 0.1 mile on Tyler Avenue to 29th Street and turn right. Continue east 0.7 mile on 29th Street and turn right into the trailhead parking lot, at the end of 29th Street. Look for the trailhead at the south end of the parking lot.

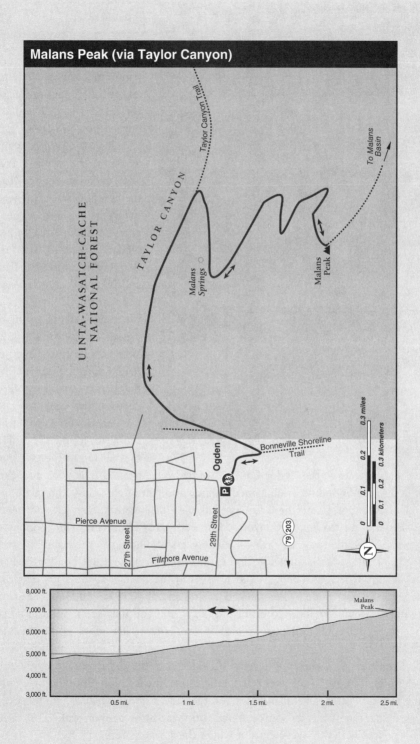

Malans Peak (via Taylor Canyon)

Taylor Canyon Trail

To Malans Basin

TAYLOR CANYON

UINTA-WASATCH-CACHE
NATIONAL FOREST

Malans
Springs

Malans
Peak

Bonneville Shoreline
Trail

Ogden

P

Pierce Avenue

27th Street

29th Street

Fillmore Avenue

79 203

0.3 miles

0.3 kilometers

0.2

0.1   0.2

0.1

0   0

N

8,000 ft.

7,000 ft.   Malans
                                                                  Peak
6,000 ft.

5,000 ft.

4,000 ft.

3,000 ft.

0.5 mi.   1 mi.   1.5 mi.   2 mi.   2.5 mi.

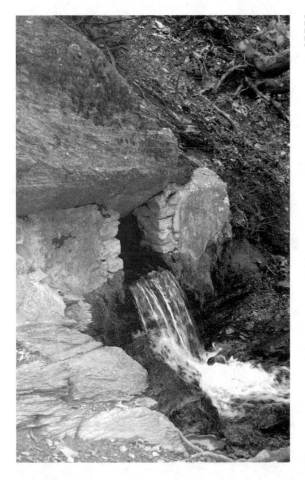

Malans Springs

panoramic views, lodging, and meals (including steak) for $6 a week. The hotel burned down in 1906.

Taylor Canyon, which leads to the Malans Peak Trail, is easily accessed from the 29th Street trailhead, which is also a popular access point for the Mount Ogden Exercise Trail, the Bonneville Shoreline Trail, and Waterfall Canyon (see next profile). Joggers and mountain bikers regularly use this network of trails. While often dry and exposed to the sun, the paths along the bench quickly lead to deep, shaded canyons.

From the 29th Street trailhead, follow the trail up the hillside to the east with the signs pointing to the Taylor Canyon South Trail. After 0.2 mile you've reached the Bonneville Shoreline Trail, gained a quick 100 feet of elevation, and taken in a good view of Ogden and the Great Salt Lake. At this junction, turn left and follow the sign leading to Taylor Canyon. After 100 yards along the wide Bonneville Shoreline Trail, the route to Taylor Canyon veers off and up to the right.

The trail leads through sage and Gambel oak into the mouth of Taylor Canyon and up a dry creekbed. At 0.6 mile from the trailhead, the path crosses a bridge to the north side of the creekbed. Soon after, you're engulfed in a beautiful canyon with conifers lining the side slopes. While you may see mountain bikers along the bench trails and even up into Taylor Canyon, few make it into this lush section of the canyon.

Continuing up the canyon, you'll notice that the dry creek suddenly runs with water, but for only about 0.2 mile along the canyon floor before going underground. After several minutes of creekside companionship, you'll see the creek descending from its source about 100 feet up the canyon wall. The creekbed is generally dry above the point where the spring enters.

About 100 feet beyond where the creek reaches the canyon floor, you'll cross a bridge over the dry creekbed. This begins a series of steep switchbacks leading up the north slope of Malans Peak. Along the ascent, you'll see the spring as it emerges from the wall of the canyon.

Continue climbing the steep, shaded slope of Gambel oak sprinkled with spruce and fir. Along the way, and in the bottom of the canyon, you may see deer and an occasional raccoon or porcupine.

At the rocky crest of Malans Peak the trees thin, opening up wide-angle views of the Great Salt Lake and peaks to the north and south. Looking back down the canyon slope, you've just ascended 1,400 vertical feet in about 1.2 miles, but the view makes every step worth it.

NEARBY ACTIVITIES

Ogden is a vibrant hub for year-round outdoor and indoor recreation. The **Salomon Center** (338 23rd St.; 801-399-5862; **salomoncenter.com**) is a high-adventure downtown sports complex with a vertical wind tunnel that simulates freefall skydiving, an indoor surf wave, and a huge climbing wall. The center also features 32 bowling lanes, billiards, a 55,000-square-foot gym, arcades, bumper cars, and restaurants.

5   WATERFALL CANYON

KEY AT-A-GLANCE INFORMATION

LENGTH: 2.6 miles round-trip

ELEVATION GAIN: 1,492'

ELEVATION AT TRAILHEAD: 4,780'

CONFIGURATION: Out-and-back

DIFFICULTY: Moderate

SCENERY: Spectacular waterfall in a deep canyon

EXPOSURE: Mostly shaded above bench trails

TRAFFIC: Busy on bench trails, moderate on upper trail

TRAIL SURFACE: Dirt and rock, becoming mostly rock near the waterfall

HIKING TIME: 1.5–2 hours

WATER REQUIREMENTS: 1 liter

SEASON: Year-round; negligible avalanche risk in Waterfall Canyon

ACCESS: On private property. No fees or permits. Trailhead parking lot and gates close at dusk.

MAPS: USGS Ogden

FACILITIES: No restrooms or water at trailhead

DOGS: On leash

SPECIAL COMMENTS: Can also be combined with Malans Peak (see previous profile) as a scenic loop hike

GPS TRAILHEAD COORDINATES

N41° 12.644´ W111° 55.917´

IN BRIEF

A beautiful hike, the Waterfall Canyon Trail follows a creek up a deep canyon to a breathtaking surprise. Area hikers love the steep, short trail, while trail runners and mountain bikers use the lower trail network, which connects the canyon with the Bonneville Shoreline Trail and other city trailheads.

DESCRIPTION

The dozens of canyons that flank the foothills of the Wasatch Front are full of surprises. Some are dry and some are wet, and you can't always be sure which is which from the valley below. As you walk along the dry bench trails above Ogden's eastern hillside, you'd never suspect a 200-foot waterfall to be spraying down a rock face just minutes up the trail.

The 29th Street trailhead provides the easiest access to Waterfall Canyon. This trailhead is also a popular access point for the Mount Ogden Exercise Trail, the Bonneville Shoreline Trail, Taylor Canyon, and Malans Peak (see previous profile).

From the 29th Street trailhead, follow the trail up the hillside to the east with the

----

Directions ⸻→

Take I-15 north from Salt Lake City to 31st Street in Ogden (Exit 341A). Go east 1.1 miles on 31st Street to Washington Boulevard (US 89) and turn left. Go north 0.1 mile to 30th Street and turn right. Continue east 1.3 miles on 30th Street to Tyler Avenue and turn left. Go north 0.1 mile on Tyler Avenue to 29th Street and turn right. Continue east 0.7 mile on 29th Street and turn right into the trailhead parking lot, at the end of 29th Street. The trailhead is at the south end of the parking lot.

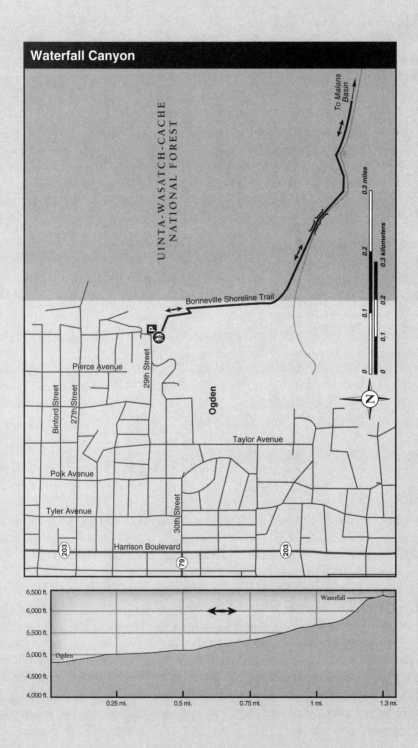

Waterfall Canyon

UINTA-WASATCH-CACHE
NATIONAL FOREST

To Malans
Basin

Bonneville Shoreline Trail

Pierce Avenue

29th Street

Binford Street

27th Street

Ogden

Taylor Avenue

Polk Avenue

30th Street

Tyler Avenue

Harrison Boulevard

203

79

203

0.3 miles

0.2

0.1

0

0.3 kilometers

0.2

0.1

0

6,500 ft.

6,000 ft.

5,500 ft.

5,000 ft.

4,500 ft.

4,000 ft.

Waterfall

Ogden

0.25 mi.   0.5 mi.   0.75 mi.   1 mi.   1.3 mi.

Mouth of Waterfall Canyon

signs pointing to the Taylor Canyon South Trail. Upon reaching the Bonneville Shoreline Trail at 0.2 mile, take a sharp right and continue south along the wide trail. This portion of the trail is often shadeless and hot in the summer.

At 0.5 mile the path turns east into Waterfall Canyon and begins a steep ascent of the northern slope of Malans Peak. After another 0.2 mile you'll come to a bridge on the right with a sign that points to Strong's Canyon. You can either cross the wooden bridge and take an immediate left or take the faint trail up the north side of the creek.

Within another 100 feet you'll pass a second bridge. Again, you can follow the trail up either side of the creek. The trails on both sides of the creek are equally beautiful and comparable in terrain. They both stay within 5–10 feet of the creek, so getting lost is never a problem.

After you cross the bridges, the trail becomes more rocky and may even become a little difficult for small children and less-agile hikers. But at this point the waterfall appears and you'll immediately forget the steep climb.

A scramble up a talus slope leads to the base of the waterfall. Its height and the narrowness of the canyon make photographing the entire waterfall almost impossible. You'll be tempted to climb the rocks on the canyon wall opposite the falls to get the perfect picture, but these crags can be dangerous. Also keep in mind that as a guest on private property, you should stay on the trail and protect the canyon's natural beauty.

If you're full of energy, make a longer scenic loop hike by climbing the steep, rocky slope to the right of the waterfall. This drainage leads up to Malans Basin, on to Malans Peak, and then down Taylor Canyon. If you make this 5-mile loop, do it counterclockwise: you can more safely ascend the rocky drainage above the waterfall than descend it.

NEARBY ACTIVITIES

Just a mile down the hillside from Waterfall Canyon, you'll find **Weber State University.** The 12,000-seat Dee Events Center hosts Weber State sports, concerts, and other campus and community events. For tickets and event information, call 801-626-6500 or visit **community.weber.edu/deeeventscenter.**

North: Davis County (Hikes 6–10)

UINTA-WASATCH-CACHE
NATIONAL FOREST

Francis Peak Road
Farmington Canyon Road
Farmington
Kaysville
Bountiful
North Salt Lake

Great Salt Lake

Antelope Island
Frary Peak

6 miles
6 kilometers

N

NORTH
(DAVIS COUNTY)

6 ADAMS CANYON

KEY AT-A-GLANCE INFORMATION

LENGTH: 3.6 miles round-trip

ELEVATION GAIN: 1,268'

ELEVATION AT TRAILHEAD: 4,832'

CONFIGURATION: Out-and-back

DIFFICULTY: Moderate

SCENERY: Valley views, deep-canyon stream, waterfall

EXPOSURE: Partially shaded initially, then mostly shaded in the canyon

TRAFFIC: Moderate

TRAIL SURFACE: Dirt, rock

HIKING TIME: 2–3 hours

WATER REQUIREMENTS: 1 liter

SEASON: Year-round

ACCESS: No fees or permits. Adams Canyon lies within Uinta-Wasatch-Cache National Forest.

MAPS: USGS Kaysville and Peterson

FACILITIES: No restrooms or water at trailhead

DOGS: On leash

SPECIAL COMMENTS: Adams Canyon is especially beautiful in late spring as the creek swells with snowmelt.

GPS TRAILHEAD COORDINATES

N41° 3.980´ W111° 54.580´

IN BRIEF

From the valley floor, Adams Canyon appears no different from any other ordinary canyon along the Wasatch Front. But once inside, you'll find a deep canyon filled with white fir, a tumbling creek, and a stunning waterfall waiting at the end of the trail.

DESCRIPTION

Locals have done a good job of keeping Adams Canyon a secret. No signs at the trailhead indicate where you are or that you can even access the canyon. The canyon's name differs from the name of the creek (North Fork Holmes Creek), which only makes it more anonymous. Even the spectacular waterfall at the end of the hike is nameless. Still, locals count this as a favorite hike, enjoying the canyon's deep-forest setting, vibrant mountain stream, and plunging waterfall.

From the northeast corner of the large parking area, take the trail leading along the fence through a thicket of Gambel oak. After 100 yards the path turns left up a steep slope and follows a series of switchbacks up the hillside. This part of the trail cuts through the sandy slopes of the Lake Bonneville shoreline

Directions

Take I-15 north from Salt Lake City to US 89/NB Ogden (Exit 324). Continue north 5.7 miles on US 89 to Oak Hills Drive. Crossing Oak Hills Drive, continue north another 0.3 mile on US 89 and turn right, onto the Eastside Drive frontage road. Continue south 0.3 mile on Eastside Drive to the trailhead parking lot, on the left. The unmarked parking area lies at the northeast corner of Eastside Drive and Canyon Creek Drive (350 North).

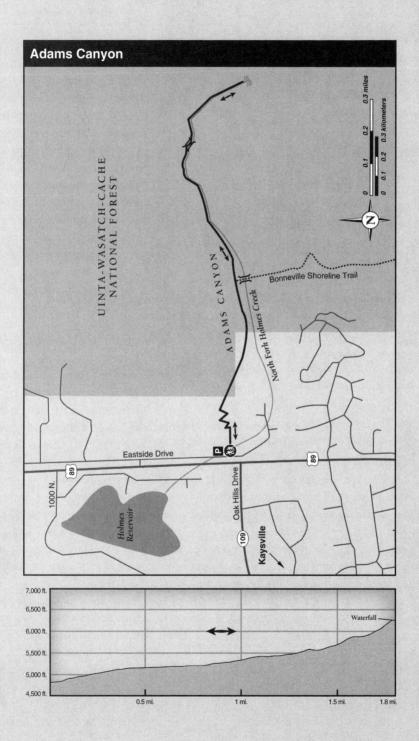

Adams Canyon

UINTA-WASATCH-CACHE NATIONAL FOREST

ADAMS CANYON

North Fork Holmes Creek

Bonneville Shoreline Trail

Eastside Drive

89

89

1000 N.

Oak Hills Drive

Holmes Reservoir

109

Kaysville

0.3 miles
0.2
0.1
0
0.3 kilometers
0.2
0.1
0

7,000 ft.
6,500 ft.
6,000 ft.
5,500 ft.
5,000 ft.
4,500 ft.

Waterfall

0.5 mi.   1 mi.   1.5 mi.   1.8 mi.

Waterfall in Adams Canyon

and is particularly prone to erosion. Stay on the trail to avoid making the problem worse. At 0.2 mile you come to a quick overlook of the Great Salt Lake with views of mountains to the north and south. This overlook demonstrates how much the view can change with just a few hundred feet of elevation gain.

Along the first part of the hike, you might well see a snake sunning itself on the trail. Frequent visitors include bull snakes, gopher snakes, and rattlers. Avoid surprising them at close range by watching the trail ahead; you can create a little noise to send them safely slithering into the underbrush. You might also glimpse deer, which often graze on the lower slopes, especially in winter.

At 0.5 mile the trail curves to the left and begins to enter the mouth of Adams Canyon. From the partially shaded slopes of oak on the north side of the canyon, you can see the towering conifers that cover its south side. Soon you become aware of the creek below on the canyon floor. At 0.7 mile another trail bends to the right and descends to a footbridge that crosses the creek. This is the Bonneville Shoreline Trail, which continues south. Stay on the trail straight ahead as it leads up Adams Canyon and along the bank of the north fork of Holmes Creek.

As you ascend the canyon, the trail steepens and becomes rockier. Holmes Creek is a fast-dropping stream with dozens of cascades and tumbles. The trail manages to parallel the creek's steep gradient as it winds around rocks and trees. White fir trees, most with trunks 2 feet in diameter, provide ample shade.

At 1.4 miles, the trail crosses from the north to the south side of the creek on a rickety wooden footbridge. Soon you pass several fire rings and primitive campsites. At one point, a huge slab of rock the size of a school bus blocks the trail as it meets the stream. Circumvent the rock most easily by climbing around on the right top side of the slab.

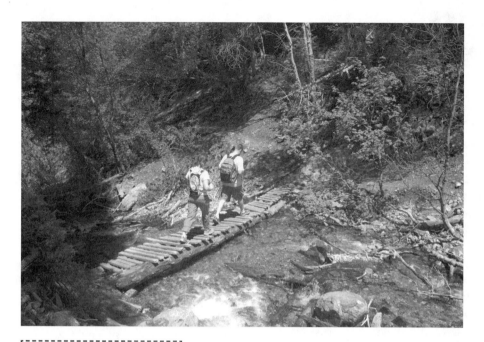

Footbridge crossing Holmes Creek

In the last 0.4 mile leading up to the waterfall, you'll find several steep sections of the creek with large cascades that could be appropriately considered waterfalls. In spring, abundant snowmelt easily triples the creek's flow, making these cascades particularly scenic. Beyond them, a bit of scrambling around rocks and tree trunks is required before arriving at the rock cliff that forms the backdrop for the waterfall. One last crossing of the creek will take you to the base of the falls, where you can enjoy the view and rest on a nearby rock or ledge. Throughout most of the year, you can easily cross the creek by stepping on large rocks, but in the surge of spring snowmelt, plan to get your feet wet.

NEARBY ACTIVITIES

Cherry Hill Water Park, Family Fun Center, and Camping Resort is off US 89 at 1325 S. Main in Kaysville, just 4 miles from the Adams Canyon trailhead. The resort features camping facilities, a water park, miniature golf, batting cages, a climbing wall, and other family-oriented activities. The campground is open year-round, while the recreational portion of the resort is open April 1–September 15. Call 888-446-2267 or visit **cherry-hill.com** for information and reservations.

7 THURSTON PEAK

 KEY AT-A-GLANCE INFORMATION

LENGTH: 8.6 miles

ELEVATION GAIN: 706'

ELEVATION AT TRAILHEAD: 9,187'

CONFIGURATION: Out-and-back

DIFFICULTY: Moderate

SCENERY: Excellent views in all directions

EXPOSURE: No shade

TRAFFIC: Light

TRAIL SURFACE: Dirt, rock

HIKING TIME: 4–5.5 hours

WATER REQUIREMENTS: 1–2 liters; no water on trail

SEASON: Late spring, summer, early fall

ACCESS: No fees or permits. Trail lies within Uinta-Wasatch-Cache National Forest.

MAPS: USGS Peterson

FACILITIES: No restrooms or water at the trailhead

DOGS: Permitted

SPECIAL COMMENTS: Most people in the valley below recognize Francis Peak by the radar installation that looks like two giant golf balls. But the higher Thurston Peak to the north is generally unknown.

GPS TRAILHEAD COORDINATES

N41° 1.663´ W111° 50.283´

IN BRIEF

Thurston Peak, at 9,706 feet, straddles the Davis–Morgan county line and is the tallest peak in each county. The ridge route from Francis Peak to Thurston Peak offers nonstop views of the valleys below and far beyond. High alpine vegetation and wildlife come together in a remote setting.

DESCRIPTION

A trail that begins at a federal radar installation and follows a dirt road for half the distance to the summit may not sound like a remote wilderness experience. And a summit that's just 519 feet higher than the trailhead elevation may not sound like the kind of challenge you'd hoped for. But the high-alpine setting, with expansive views every step of the way, quickly erases any prejudices you may have brought to the hike. The section of trail from Francis Peak to Thurston Peak is also part of the Great Western Trail, a continuous corridor of trails that stretches from Canada to Mexico and traverses some of the most spectacular scenery in the

----

Directions ———————————————→

Take I-15 north from Salt Lake City to Farmington (Exit 322) and continue north 0.6 mile to State Street (UT 106). Turn right and go east 0.2 mile to Main Street. Turn left on Main Street and continue north 0.6 mile to 600 North. Turn left on 600 North, continue east 0.1 mile to 100 East, and turn left. Continue north on 100 East as it turns into Farmington Canyon Road. Continue 8 miles up Farmington Canyon Road to a junction with two gates. Drive through the left gate and follow the road 4.3 miles to the locked gate below the Francis Peak radar installation. Park on the side of the road below the gate.

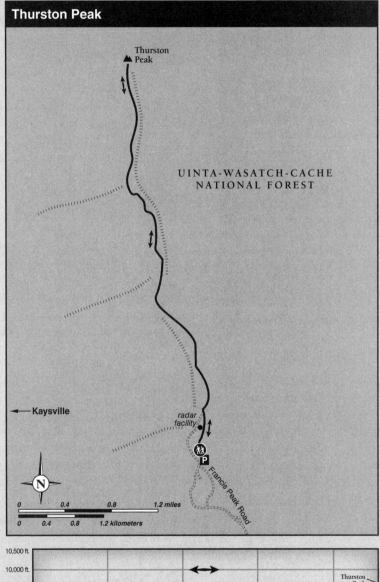

Thurston Peak

Thurston
Peak

UINTA-WASATCH-CACHE
NATIONAL FOREST

← Kaysville

radar
facility

Francis Peak Road

N

| 0 | 0.4 | 0.8 | 1.2 miles |

| 0 | 0.4 | 0.8 | 1.2 kilometers |

10,500 ft.

10,000 ft.

9,500 ft.

Francis
Peak

Thurston
Peak

9,000 ft.

8,500 ft.

8,000 ft.

1 mi.   2 mi.   3 mi.   4 mi.   4.3 mi.

Summit monument on
Thurston Peak

West (for another section of the GWT, see Hike 32, page 145).

From the locked gate on the road leading up to the radar installation at the top of Francis Peak (elevation 9,547 feet), take the dirt road to the right that follows the more level contour along the eastern slope of Francis Peak. This road stays close to the ridge for much of the way, although it generally skirts the smaller peaks by taking a gentler route along the western slopes, favoring the Davis County side.

Once the road ends, a narrow trail continues along the ridgeline. Rather than ascending each of the small, unnamed peaks along the way, it dips along the slope to an elevation as low as 9,000 feet. Even though the maximum elevation gain is only 706 feet, the repeated ups and downs produce a cumulative gain of about 3,000 feet—certainly a good workout for a round-trip hike of less than 10 miles.

The slopes are largely covered with sage and dotted with wind-mangled subalpine fir and limber pine. In the late spring and early summer, wildflowers appear as fast as the snow can melt. Large snowdrifts generally cover the slopes throughout the spring and occasionally into July. Although you'll find no precipitous drop-offs, expect to traverse some steep slopes and approach potentially unstable snow cornices with caution.

The saddle immediately south of Thurston Peak is at an elevation just under 9,100 feet, one of the lower levels of the entire trail. At this point the trail skirts Thurston Peak's western slope and continues north. To reach the summit, leave the main trail and either find a poorly defined trail or make your own way for the remaining 0.3 mile. Pink-and-black marbled granite, which composes the summit, also dots this slope.

Radar installation on Francis Peak

The wildlife along the ridge, like that of other high-alpine regions, includes marmots and cliff swallows that nest in the rocky outcrops. Deer graze in the higher meadows and slopes in the summer, and butterflies abound in the spring.

A granite marker and plaque at the summit honor Thomas Jefferson Thurston, who first viewed the Morgan Valley to the east in 1852. The inspiring view led him to build a wagon road through Weber Canyon to access Morgan Valley, where he settled in 1855. The views from the summit are breathtaking in all directions, extending far beyond the valleys and the Great Salt Lake to distant mountains and ranges to the east and west.

NEARBY ACTIVITIES

The **Farmington Bay Waterfowl Management Area** offers excellent bird-watching and biking trails. More than 200 species of waterfowl, songbirds, and raptors visit this area during the migration and nesting season. Nesting begins in early March for Canada geese and great blue herons; bald eagles winter in the area. The main entrance is southwest of Farmington at 1325 W. Glover Lane. Open 8 a.m.–5 p.m. daily; call 801-451-7386 or visit **wildlife.utah.gov/habitat/farmington_bay.php** for more information.

8   FARMINGTON CREEK TRAIL

 KEY AT-A-GLANCE INFORMATION

LENGTH: 3.2 miles round-trip

ELEVATION GAIN: 1,178'

ELEVATION: 5,245' (Farmington Creek), 6,423' (Sunset Campground)

CONFIGURATION: Out-and-back or one-way with shuttle

DIFFICULTY: Moderate

SCENERY: Canyon views, stream, waterfall

EXPOSURE: Mostly sunny

TRAFFIC: Light

TRAIL SURFACE: Dirt, rock

HIKING TIME: 2.5–3 hours round-trip

WATER REQUIREMENTS: 1–1.5 liters

SEASON: Best in spring and fall

ACCESS: No fees or permits. Trail lies within Uinta-Wasatch-Cache National Forest.

MAPS: USGS Bountiful Peak, Peterson

FACILITIES: No restrooms or water at trailhead; vault toilet at Sunset Campground

DOGS: On leash

SPECIAL COMMENTS: Farmington Creek Trail is also called the Sunset Trail, since it ends at the Sunset Campground.

GPS TRAILHEAD COORDINATES

Farmington Creek (lower trailhead):
N41° 0.018´ W111° 51.983´

Sunset Campground (upper trailhead):
N41° 0.137´ W111° 50.400´

IN BRIEF

The trail follows Farmington Creek, the largest stream or river in Davis County, up a broad canyon to a primitive U.S. Forest Service campground. A 40-foot waterfall near the top of the trail and expansive views make Farmington Canyon a rewarding destination, especially in spring and fall.

DESCRIPTION

Farmington Creek cuts through a wide canyon fed by several tributary creeks and springs. By the time it reaches the lower canyon, the water flow is substantial enough that it's probably outgrown its simple creek designation. The Farmington Creek Trail ascends steadily along the south slope of the canyon, providing great views of the canyon and the creek below. Although the road above the trail receives year-round recreational use by ATVs, snowmobiles, and hunters, the trail below remains relatively quiet.

At the lower trailhead, take either of the steep trails at the north end of the small

---

Directions ⟶

Take I-15 north from Salt Lake City to Farmington (Exit 322) and continue north 0.6 mile to State Street. Turn right and go east 0.2 mile to Main Street (UT 106). Turn left on Main Street and continue north 0.6 mile to 600 North. Turn right on 600 North, continue east 0.1 mile to 100 East, and turn left. Continue north on 100 East as it turns into Farmington Canyon Road. Continue 1.6 miles up Farmington Canyon Road to a dirt parking area on the right, at the point where the pavement ends. Sunset Campground, the upper end of the trail, is another 5 miles up Farmington Canyon Road (and a handy spot to park a second car if you want to make this a one-way hike).

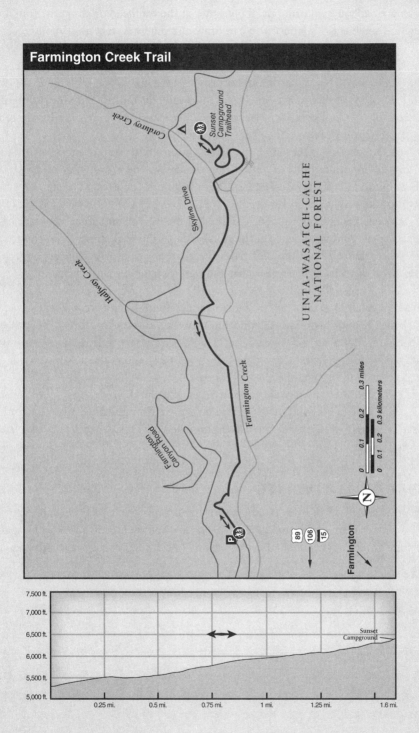

Farmington Creek Trail

Corduroy Creek

Sunset Campground Trailhead

Skyline Drive

Halfway Creek

UINTA-WASATCH-CACHE NATIONAL FOREST

Farmington Creek

Farmington Canyon Road

0.3 miles

0.2   0.3 kilometers

0.1

0   0.1   0.2

0   0.1   0.2

89 106 15

Farmington

7,500 ft.
7,000 ft.
6,500 ft.   Sunset
6,000 ft.   Campground
5,500 ft.
5,000 ft.
        0.25 mi.   0.5 mi.   0.75 mi.   1 mi.   1.25 mi.   1.6 mi.

parking area. You won't find drinking water at the trailhead or along the trail, but there are small springs where you can draw and purify water. You can also access Farmington Creek at the trailhead and near the falls.

The hike follows the creek's gradient and stays 100–200 feet above the creek most of the way. The trail is on the north side of the creek, and with the exception of a few stands of oak, hikers are exposed to sunlight most of the way. Along the 1.6-mile trail, you'll cross at least four small creeks and springs as they descend into Farmington Creek.

During the spring, Farmington Creek gushes with water, and even though the trail is often hundreds of yards from the creek, you can always hear its roar below. In the fall, the flow is reduced, but the autumn colors and cooler air make for an equally pleasant hike.

Deer and foxes are frequently sighted in the canyon and along the trail. Also watch for two old cars—one on the north side of the trail, another on the south side—that plunged over the cliff from the road above nearly 50 years ago, and have made the thick underbrush near the trail their final rusting place.

At 1.3 miles the trail comes within 50 feet of the creek, near the base of a broad waterfall. A steep spur trail enables sure-footed hikers to access the creek below the 40-foot waterfall. Beyond the waterfall, the trail ascends a steep slope to the north by a series of switchbacks and, within 0.3 mile, arrives at Sunset Campground. The Farmington Creek Trail (#1621) enters the southwest side of the campground on one of the small loops.

Although there is no water at Sunset Campground, you can enjoy the shade and a snack at one of the picnic tables before returning. And if you've planned ahead, you may even have a car waiting to take you back down to the mouth of the canyon.

NEARBY ACTIVITIES

Lagoon, just off I-15 in Farmington, is the largest amusement park in Utah, with 47 rides, a water park, a historic Pioneer Village, live entertainment, shops, games, and restaurants. For a schedule and events, call 801-451-8000 or visit **lagoonpark.com.**

FRARY PEAK 9

IN BRIEF

Ascend to the summit of the largest island in the Great Salt Lake. You'll find spectacular vistas and excellent wildlife-viewing in a surprisingly distinctive geologic zone and natural habitat. This hike offers the best chance in Utah of spotting bighorn sheep.

DESCRIPTION

At only 6,596 feet in elevation, Frary Peak really isn't that remarkable by Utah standards. But it may be the most unusual summit in the state. On Antelope Island in the Great Salt Lake, the peak rises 2,400 feet above the surrounding salt flats. Its location was intriguing enough that Kit Carson and John C. Fremont made the first Anglo exploration of the island in 1845. The entire island is a high-desert grassland that provides a hospitable habitat for migrating birds, bighorn sheep, pronghorn antelope, and a herd of more than 500 bison.

You'll find the trail consistently well marked and easy to follow. From the trailhead it winds its way quickly up the island's

----

Directions ———————————————➤

Take I-15 north from Salt Lake City to Syracuse (Exit 332). At the off-ramp, turn left (west) and take UT 108 (known locally as Antelope Drive or 1700 South) west 6.7 miles to the Antelope Island entrance gate. Continue along the 6.8-mile causeway (UT 127) to Antelope Island. Once on the island, veer left at the RANCH sign and continue 0.6 mile to Garr Ranch Road. Turn left on Garr Ranch Road and continue 5.2 miles down the east side of the island. Turn right at the FRARY TRAILHEAD sign. Follow this paved road 0.5 mile up the island's eastern slope to the large dirt parking area. The trailhead is at the parking lot's southwest corner.

KEY AT-A-GLANCE INFORMATION

LENGTH: 6.6 miles round-trip

ELEVATION GAIN: 2,068'

ELEVATION AT TRAILHEAD: 4,528'

CONFIGURATION: Out-and-back

DIFFICULTY: Moderate

SCENERY: Superb 360-degree summit views of Great Salt Lake, valley, and surrounding peaks

EXPOSURE: No shade

TRAFFIC: Moderate

TRAIL SURFACE: Dirt, rock

HIKING TIME: 3.5–6 hours

WATER REQUIREMENTS: 1–2 liters depending on weather; no water on trail

SEASON: Generally year-round, but check for seasonal closures by calling 801-725-9263. Snow may cover trail in winter.

ACCESS: September 15–April 14, 9 a.m.–5 p.m.; April 15–September 14, 9 a.m.–6 p.m. Pay entrance fee of $9/vehicle at the state-park gate before crossing the causeway.

MAPS: USGS Antelope Island, Antelope Island North

FACILITIES: No restrooms or water at trailhead; nearest public facilities are at park visitor center, 7 miles north of trailhead

DOGS: Prohibited

GPS TRAILHEAD COORDINATES

N40° 59.623´ W112° 12.152´

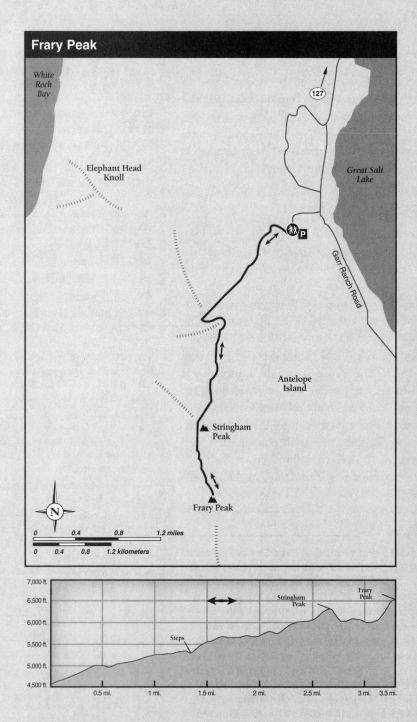

Frary Peak

grassy eastern slopes. Don't be intimidated by the first mile's steep terrain, since the trail climbs more gradually once you hit the ridgeline. At 0.7 mile you'll pass the Dooley Knob Trail junction and arrive at the island ridgeline for first views to the west.

From this lower ridgeline, the trail crosses to the island's western side and follows a fairly gentle contour along the western slopes for most of the way to the summit. As the trail begins to descend the slope and move toward the prominent Elephant Head knoll on the western shore, you might even begin to wonder if you're on the right trail. Soon, at 1.2 miles, you'll see a set of wooden steps that lead up and to the east through the rocky escarpment. These steps quickly bring you back to the ridgeline and some expansive views to both the east and west. The trail continues through grassy meadows to cross the rounded slopes of Stringham Peak (elevation 6,374 feet), capped by a large communications tower.

From Stringham Peak you have a clear view of the craggy Frary Peak summit, just 0.6 mile and about 15 minutes ahead to the south. At this point you might be tempted to follow the faint trail along the ridgeline straight ahead, but you're really much better off staying on the main trail as it descends to the right along the western slopes, losing about 150 feet of elevation. You'll soon regain the elevation loss by climbing a long flight of wooden steps that leads back up to the ridge.

The higher slopes are blanketed with big sagebrush and an occasional juniper tree, not large enough to create much shade. A short scramble up a steep slope soon brings you to the rocky, beige outcrop that is Frary Peak. The summit's flat rock provides an ideal place to sit down, enjoy lunch, and take in the views in all directions. Directly to the west, Bountiful Peak and the Wasatch Range are reflected in the Great Salt Lake. Forty miles to the southwest, you'll spot the easily recognizable Deseret Peak (11,031 feet). On a clear day, you can even see Ibapah Peak (12,087 feet) nearly 120 miles to the southwest.

The rocky slopes near the summit also provide a good place to watch for bighorn sheep. The Utah Department of Wildlife introduced a herd of 22 bighorn to the island in 1996, as a nursery herd that could supply animals to other areas of the state. With few natural predators, the bighorn population on the island has grown to 160, and portions of the herd are frequently exported. If you don't happen to see a bighorn, you'll certainly see their clumps of wool along the trail.

Nearly 200 pronghorn antelope and 350 deer graze the island's slopes and rangelands. But Antelope Island's most famous residents are the bison, often found grazing along the trail. The 12 animals introduced in 1893 as part of a private ranch and hunting preserve formed the foundation for today's free-roaming herd of 500–700.

Antelope Island plays host to millions of migratory birds each year. The Great Salt Lake's brine flies and brine shrimp provide a primary food source for many of the area's 250 bird species.

Along the trail you'll often spot western meadowlarks, yellow-headed blackbirds, and various raptors. Chukars nest year-round on the island, concealed in rocks or in the brush near the trail.

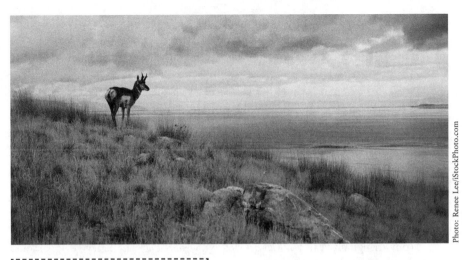

Photo: Renee Lee/iStockPhoto.com

An antelope gazes over the Great Salt Lake.

Although you'll find no water on the trail, Antelope Island's 40 major fresh-water springs, primarily on the eastern slopes, produce 36 million gallons of water annually and support much of the island's wildlife and vegetation. The island's geology exposes some of the oldest rocks on Earth in the 2.7-billion-year-old Farmington Canyon complex. Along the trail you'll also see granite, limestone outcrops, and shale.

Range grasses such as purple threeawn cover most of the lower meadows and slopes. Common wildflowers along the trail include fiddleneck, a bristly annual with yellow flowers, and the vernal daisy.

Frary Peak is an ideal hike in the early spring when most of the higher moun-tain trails are still covered in snow. Summer can be grueling on the shadeless trail, so bring plenty of water. Fall brings more pleasant hiking conditions, along with migrating raptors, pronghorn harems, and more-frequent buck deer sightings. Throughout the year, Frary Peak offers exceptional views surrounded by a sur-prising and continually varying array of wildlife.

NEARBY ACTIVITIES

The **Antelope Island State Park Visitor Center,** at the island's north end, is open year-round (801-725-9263). Here you'll find exhibits, a bookstore, restrooms, and a video presentation on the island's natural and human history. Knowledgeable rangers provide interpretive assistance and suggestions on wildlife-viewing. Popu-lar events offered throughout the year center around bird migrations and the annual bison roundup. Look for the day-use facility and primitive campgrounds on the north side of the island. The day-use area offers covered picnic tables, drinking water, restrooms, and showers for those wanting to take a dip in the Great Salt Lake's buoyant water.

KENNY CREEK TRAIL 10

IN BRIEF

This steep trail follows three separate mountain springs through deep woods and open meadows, finally arriving at a 100-year-old miner's cabin. The trail is as popular with deer and moose as it is with humans.

DESCRIPTION

Some trails switchback or wind their way up the side of a mountain to mitigate the steep ascent, but not the Kenny Creek Trail. The miners who worked this area 100 years ago found the most direct means possible to reach their lode, and the Kenny Creek Trail is it. In less than 2.2 miles you gain more than 2,200 feet without ever having to scramble or use your hands.

The Kenny Creek Trail starts on the north side of the road, across from the parking area and restrooms in Bountiful's Mueller Park. While Mueller Park is a popular mountain-biking destination, most mountain bikers find the Kenny Park Trail too steep and narrow for biking pleasure.

From Mueller Park Road, the trail ascends through dense woods along the western bank of Kenny Creek. Even during spring runoff,

KEY AT-A-GLANCE INFORMATION

LENGTH: 4.5 miles round-trip
ELEVATION GAIN: 2,217'
ELEVATION AT TRAILHEAD: 5,247'
CONFIGURATION: Out-and-back
DIFFICULTY: Moderate
SCENERY: Valley views, creeks, spring-fed mountain meadows
EXPOSURE: Mostly shaded
TRAFFIC: Light
TRAIL SURFACE: Dirt
HIKING TIME: 2.5–3.5 hours
WATER REQUIREMENTS: 1–2 liters
SEASON: Spring, summer, fall
ACCESS: Fee of $2 payable at Mueller Park Entrance. Gate closes at 10 p.m.
MAPS: USGS Fort Douglas
FACILITIES: Restrooms and water at the trailhead parking area
DOGS: On leash
SPECIAL COMMENTS: With thick underbrush and a narrow trail, you'll want long pants on this hike.

Directions

Take I-15 north from Salt Lake City to 2600 South in Bountiful (Exit 315). At the off-ramp, turn right and go east on 2600 South. After 1 mile, 2600 South curves to the left and becomes Orchard Drive. Continue north on Orchard Drive to 1800 South and turn right (1.7 miles from the I-15 exit). Continue east 2.2 miles on 1800 South, which becomes Mueller Park Road, to the Mueller Park entrance. Enter the first parking area on the right. You'll find the trailhead across the street.

GPS TRAILHEAD COORDINATES

N40° 51.790´ W111° 50.053´

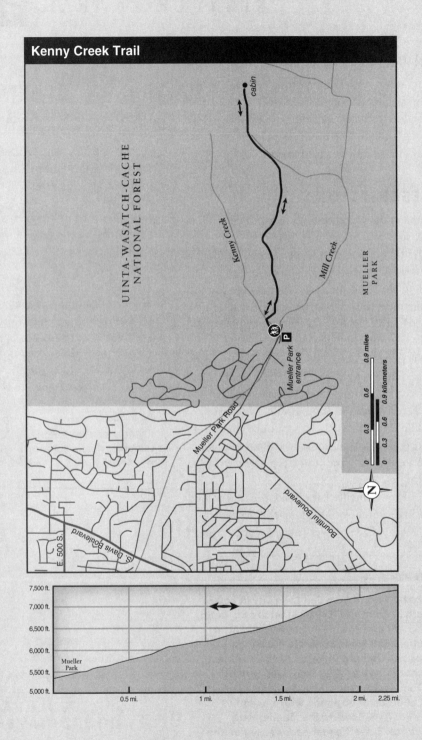

Kenny Creek Trail

cabin

UINTA-WASATCH-CACHE
NATIONAL FOREST

Kenny Creek

Mill Creek

MUELLER
PARK

Mueller Park
entrance

P

Mueller Park Road

Bountiful Boulevard

S. Davis Boulevard

E. 500 S.

0.9 miles
0.6
0.3
0

0.9 kilometers
0.6
0.3
0

N

7,500 ft.
7,000 ft.
6,500 ft.
6,000 ft.
5,500 ft.
5,000 ft.

Mueller
Park

0.5 mi.   1 mi.   1.5 mi.   2 mi.   2.25 mi.

Ruins of miner's cabin on Kenny Creek Trail

Kenny Creek is only a few feet wide and can easily be stepped across without getting your feet wet. After the trail crosses Kenny Creek at 0.2 mile, you won't see it again until your return.

After leaving the creek, the trail ascends quickly through a ground cover of grasses, forbs, and mountain shrubs under the shade of oak and maple. The trail is narrow, and the thick chaparral will scrape unprotected legs to pieces. Wear long pants and save your legs for another hike.

At 0.9 mile, the trail leaves Mueller Park and enters Uinta-Wasatch-Cache National Forest. The forest canopy opens briefly to display views of the Great Salt Lake, Antelope Island, and mountains to the west. But even at this overlook, you'll notice hillside homes across the canyon at the same elevation. It will take more climbing to escape encroaching development.

As the trail rises above the meadow, you encounter a large thicket of Gambel oak. You'll swear you're bushwhacking, but a trail actually exists under the brush. It's maintained but intentionally preserved as an unimproved wilderness trail.

The path crosses perennial streams and meadows between stands of oak and maple. At higher elevations, above 7,300 feet, clusters of quaking aspen dot the hillside. Moose and deer inhabit these higher slopes year-round and use the trail regularly. Watch for their tracks on the wet trail, along with those of mountain lions. In the trees, spotted towhees and mountain chickadees make their nests.

After 2.2 miles of heart-pounding ascent, you'll come to an old miner's cabin in a clearing: a great place to take a rest and consider your options. Most hikers

Photo: DoxaDigital/iStockPhoto.com

Buffalo on Antelope Island

make the cabin their destination and turnaround point, but you can also climb the higher ridge in the Sessions Mountains to the northeast and access the Great Western Trail, or head to the southeast along a faint and sometimes nonexistent trail to Willey Hollow. If you choose to turn around at the cabin, you've given your legs and your heart a great workout and you'll enjoy the speedy descent.

NEARBY ACTIVITIES

Mueller Park is within minutes of Bountiful neighborhoods and shopping areas. For mountain bikers, the Mueller Park Trail is a great lower-altitude alpine ride that can be done as a 7-mile route to Big Rock or a 13-mile out-and-back to Rudy's Flat. Restrooms, water, and picnic facilities are available.

Photo: Rob Witt

Central: Salt Lake County (Hikes 11–42)

City Creek

Red Butte Creek

East Canyon Creek

11

12

65

EMIGRATION CANYON

Salt Lake City
13
14
15

15

80

16
Summit Park

PARLEYS CANYON

17

71

89

186

South Salt Lake

80

19
20
18

21
22

23

MILL CREEK CANYON

266

Mount Olympus

25 26
27
28

30

24

190

29

BIG COTTONWOOD CANYON

Brighton
32

215

Cottonwood Heights

Alta
33 34
35
36

31

209

40

37 38
39

42

89

210

LITTLE COTTONWOOD CANYON

UINTA-WASATCH-CACHE
NATIONAL FOREST

15
Draper

Lone Peak

41

N

0   2   4   6 miles

0   2   4   6 kilometers

CENTRAL
(SALT LAKE COUNTY)

11 MORMON PIONEER TRAIL

KEY AT-A-GLANCE INFORMATION

LENGTH: 9.1 miles one-way

ELEVATION GAIN: 1,364'

ELEVATION: 6,039' (Mormon Flat), 5,796' (Little Dell Reservoir), 7,403' (Big Mountain Pass)

CONFIGURATION: One-way as described (but see Directions)

DIFFICULTY: Moderate

SCENERY: Canyon drainage, mountain views, view of Salt Lake Valley

EXPOSURE: Mostly shaded

TRAFFIC: Moderate

TRAIL SURFACE: Dirt, some rocks

HIKING TIME: 4–5 hours

WATER REQUIREMENTS: 2 liters

SEASON: Late spring, summer, early fall

ACCESS: No fees for access or parking at Mormon Flat. Seasonal parking fees charged at Little Dell Reservoir. Gate to Big Mountain and Mormon Flat closes during winter.

MAPS: USGS Mountain Dell

FACILITIES: Restrooms at both trailheads and at Big Mountain and Affleck Park. No drinking water at trailheads.

DOGS: Prohibited in Mountain Dell Canyon

GPS TRAILHEAD COORDINATES

Mormon Flat:
N40° 48.930´ W111° 35.090´

Little Dell Reservoir:
N40° 46.620´ W111° 41.318´

Big Mountain Pass:
N40° 49.680´ W111° 39.218´

IN BRIEF

The Donner Party blazed this historic trail in 1846, followed by 70,000 Mormon pioneers from 1847 to 1868. The trail also served as a leg of the Pony Express route. Still, for all its history, this section of the trail remains an inviting, tranquil, and exceptionally beautiful path through the woods of a gentle canyon. It's most alluring in late spring and early fall.

If you can do only a short portion of the hike or a round-trip, choose the quieter, more remote 4-mile section from Mormon Flat to Big Mountain, where your chances of sharing the trail with wildlife are increased.

DESCRIPTION

As the Mormon pioneers began their epic 1,300-mile trek from Nauvoo, Illinois, to the Salt Lake Valley, they didn't know that the steepest and longest sustained ascent—and the highest elevation of the entire journey—would occur at the end of the trail, on the day they first glimpsed their destination. This historic section of the Mormon Pioneer Trail captures that last full day of the trip and gives modern hikers some sense of what it might have been like to be a pioneer on a westward journey.

The 9.1-mile section of the trail was originally blazed by the ill-fated Donner Party in 1846, a year before the Mormon pioneers came along. It took the Donner Party's 87 members more than a week to cut a road through the underbrush that you will hike in 5 hours or less. That delay would prove disastrous, as the party was caught in a winter storm in the Sierra Nevada less than three months later.

California gold-seekers and the Overland Stage used the trail in the 1850s. In 1860 and

Mormon Pioneer Trail

Big Mountain

65

Big Mountain
Pass Trailhead

Big Mountain
Pass

Mormon
Flat

AFFLECK
PARK

East Canyon Creek

East Canyon Road

65

Bald Mountain

Little Dell
Trailhead

Little Dell
Reservoir

UINTA-WASATCH-CACHE
NATIONAL FOREST

80

80

N

0   0.5   1   1.5 miles

0   0.5   1   1.5 kilometers

Big
Mountain

8,000 ft.

7,500 ft.

7,000 ft.

6,500 ft.

Mormon
Flat

Affleck
Park

6,000 ft.

5,500 ft.

2 mi.   4 mi.   6 mi.   8 mi.   9.1 mi.

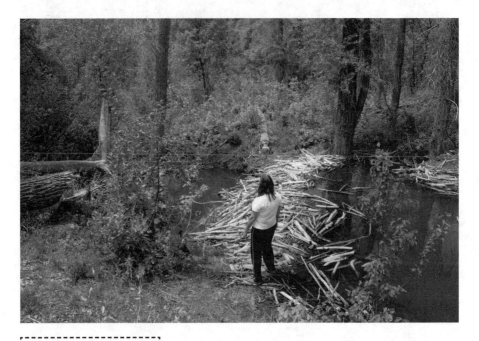

Beaver dam at Affleck Park

Directions

The Mormon Pioneer Trail is best enjoyed as a one-way hike re-creating the arrival of the pioneers as they traveled from Mormon Flat up to Big Mountain Pass, where they first saw the Salt Lake Valley, and down into Mountain Dell Canyon. The one-way hike requires leaving a shuttle vehicle at Little Dell. The hike can also be done in shorter one-way or round-trip segments, using Big Mountain Pass as a stopping or turnaround point.

MORMON FLAT (starting trailhead): Take I-80 east from Salt Lake City to Jeremy Ranch (Exit 143). Turn left at the off-ramp, cross under I-80, and turn left onto Rasmussen Road. Continue 0.1 mile to Jeremy Ranch Road and turn right. Continue 4.2 miles on Jeremy Ranch Road up East Canyon to the Mormon Flat parking area, on the left. Cross the footbridge over East Canyon Creek to the well-marked trailhead.

LITTLE DELL RESERVOIR (ending trailhead): Take I-80 east from Salt Lake City to the Emigration and East Canyons (UT 65, Exit 134). Turn left and proceed north 3 miles on UT 65 to the Little Dell Recreation Area parking lot, on the right. The trail can be accessed from the east end of the parking area, near the reservoir's shore.

BIG MOUNTAIN PASS (trail midpoint and alternate trailhead): From the Little Dell Recreation Area parking lot, continue east 5 miles on UT 65 up Mountain Dell Canyon to the large Big Mountain Pass parking area, on the right. The trail to Mormon Flat departs down the slope on the lot's east side, while the trail to Little Dell begins from the lot's southwest side.

1861, the trail served as the Pony Express route through the Wasatch Mountains. Riders would leave Bauchmann's Station (now covered by East Canyon Reservoir) on East Canyon Creek and arrive at the Mountain Dell Station within several hours.

To recapture the lore and scenic appeal of this historic trail, leave a shuttle vehicle at Little Dell Reservoir (the trail's end), then drive on to Mormon Flat on East Canyon Creek. Cross the creek through a meadow of low-lying willow, and follow the trail as it enters the mouth of Little Emigration Canyon—you're immediately transported back more than 150 years.

Within 0.5 mile after entering the canyon, the trail joins with a cottonwood-lined creek. The trail gradually ascends the wide canyon floor, which is marked with aspen and spruce. Pioneers would have welcomed the shade of the wooded slopes, having just spent much of their journey on the open plains of Nebraska and Wyoming. Like you, they may have seen their first moose or beaver dam while walking through this lush drainage. They also may have spotted a cougar or been lucky enough to augment their diminishing rations with some venison.

At 3.5 miles, the trail steepens as it approaches Big Mountain Pass, gaining about 400 feet of elevation in the final 0.5 mile. When you arrive at the pass (now a parking lot with restrooms and a historical marker), take a moment to gaze to the west and imagine what it would have been like to have walked more than 1,300 miles and suddenly see your ultimate destination laid out below. On July 23, 1847, Brigham Young arrived at this pass, gazed out over the Salt Lake Valley, and said, "This is the place. Drive on." Three days earlier, Orson Pratt had arrived at Big Mountain Pass and measured the elevation at 7,245 feet above sea level. Although the actual elevation is 7,403 feet, his calculation was amazingly accurate given the simple handheld instruments of the day.

From Big Mountain Pass, the party locked their wagon wheels with chains, attached a drag shoe, and essentially slid down the slope into Mountain Dell Canyon, arriving near Affleck Park, where they camped for the night. Your Big Mountain descent will be less treacherous on a singletrack trail that switchbacks down the head of the canyon through groves of aspen, bigtooth maple, and fir. Within 1.3 miles of the pass, the trail joins Mountain Dell Creek, which continues near the trail until it enters Little Dell Reservoir. Along the way, the trail crosses the road twice and passes through Affleck Park at 2.5 miles from Big Mountain Pass, with restrooms, campsites, and picnic sites under the shade of towering cottonwoods.

Just down the trail from Affleck Park, you'll notice a small, rounded peak to the west known as Little Mountain. The pioneers camped at the base of Little Mountain before crossing into Emigration Canyon to the west and entering the Salt Lake Valley the next day. While there is a good trail leading over to Emigration Canyon from Affleck Park, the National Historic Trail follows the creek for another 1.6 miles into the Little Dell Recreation Area, where your shuttle vehicle awaits.

Note: Although road access is closed in winter, this is a popular snowshoeing and backcountry-skiing destination with a negligible avalanche hazard.

NEARBY ACTIVITIES

To complete your experience on the Mormon Pioneer Trail, visit **This Is The Place Heritage Park,** an outdoor living-history attraction that presents the story of everyday life in a typical Utah settlement from 1847 to 1897. The park includes more than 40 re-created and original buildings from settlements throughout Utah. Historically costumed staff demonstrate life as it would have been for 19th-century Utahns. The park is at the mouth of Emigration Canyon, at 2601 E. Sunnyside Ave. Call 801-582-1847 or visit **thisistheplace.org.**

EMIGRATION CANYON
MINERS TRAIL

IN BRIEF

An old jeep road, once used by fruitless prospectors and long since overgrown, leads into a hidden side canyon now frequented by knowing bow-hunters. The trail concludes at a ridgeline saddle with views into neighboring Red Butte Canyon and the Salt Lake Valley beyond.

DESCRIPTION

Salt Lake City's original hiking destination was Emigration Canyon, although you wouldn't know that today. In 1846 the Donner Party blazed the trail through Emigration Canyon from Little Mountain Summit down to the valley floor. A year later, the first company of Mormon pioneers, led by Brigham Young, would descend into the Salt Lake Valley through Emigration Canyon, which remained the primary route into the valley until the road through Parleys Canyon (now the route of Interstate 80) was completed in 1850.

In spite of its proximity to the University of Utah and downtown Salt Lake City, Emigration Canyon has retained its bucolic feel. It's still a popular training ride or day tour for local cyclists. But you don't have to stray very far from the canyon road to find quiet trails and side canyons that are no different today than they were in the 1850s.

- -

Directions ⟶

Take I-80 east of Salt Lake City to the East Canyon turnoff (Exit 134). At the end of the off-ramp, turn left and continue north 2.4 miles on UT 65 to Emigration Canyon Road. Turn left and follow the winding road 3.1 miles to the floor of Emigration Canyon. At the junction, turn right and continue 1.7 miles up Burr's Lane to the small parking area, on the left.

KEY AT-A-GLANCE INFORMATION

LENGTH: 5 miles round-trip

ELEVATION GAIN: 810'

ELEVATION AT TRAILHEAD: 6,404'

CONFIGURATION: Out-and-back

DIFFICULTY: Moderate

SCENERY: Canyon and valley views

EXPOSURE: Mostly shaded

TRAFFIC: Light

TRAIL SURFACE: Dirt, rock

HIKING TIME: 2.5–3 hours

WATER REQUIREMENTS: 1–2 liters

SEASON: Late spring, summer, fall; snowshoeing in winter

ACCESS: No fees or permits. The trail lies within Uinta-Wasatch-Cache National Forest.

MAPS: USGS Mountain Dell

FACILITIES: No restrooms or water at trailhead

DOGS: On leash

GPS TRAILHEAD COORDINATES

N40° 48.457´ W111° 43.381´

Emigration Canyon Miners Trail

UINTA-WASATCH-CACHE
NATIONAL FOREST

Killyon Canyon

Pinecrest Canyon Road

Burr Fork

Killyons Canyon Lane

Henderson Spring

Freeze Creek

Brigham Fork

Burr Lane

Emigration Canyon

Emigration Canyon Road

65

65

N

| 0 | 0.2 | 0.4 | 0.6 miles |
| 0 | 0.2 | 0.4 | 0.6 kilometers |

8,000 ft.
7,500 ft.
7,000 ft.
6,500 ft.
6,000 ft.
5,500 ft.

Ridgeline

0.5 mi.   1 mi.   1.5 mi.   2 mi.   2.5 mi.

This Is The Place Monument, at the mouth of Emigration Canyon

If you're approaching the trailhead from I-80 and UT 65 (as described in the Directions), you'll have passed Little Dell Reservoir, which fills the mouth of Mountain Dell Canyon. The first wagon trains rolled down this canyon, then climbed the slopes to the west leading to Little Mountain Summit. From there they made the crossing and descent into Emigration Canyon. Thirteen years later, a Pony Express station was built near the upper end of Little Dell Reservoir and became the last stop before Salt Lake City.

From the small roadside parking area, marked by a sign reading ARCHERY HUNTING ONLY, walk past the metal gate to the south. Continue along the wide trail, dotted on both sides with white fir, that parallels the canyon road below. At 0.3 mile the trail divides—stay to the right. At 0.6 mile the trail follows the contour of the hillside and begins a sweeping curve to the west, into a quiet unmarked canyon known as Brigham Fork.

A gentle ascent up the east side of Brigham Fork brings you to outcroppings of red sandstone first noticeable about 1.5 miles from the trailhead. This is the same vein of red sandstone that appears in various canyons throughout the Wasatch and that gives Red Butte Canyon (immediately to the west) its name. Soon the trail steepens and becomes rocky, with bursts of sandstone.

Now deep in Brigham Fork and 2.1 miles from the trailhead, you'll step across a small creek in the canyon hollow and begin ascending steeply through

mature stands of white pine. Passing through a small meadow often used by hunters and backcountry campers, the trail curves left and to the west as it makes its
way toward the ridgeline.

As you make your way up to the ridgeline saddle, notice the tender bent
aspens on the slope. With its low elevations and lack of shade, the ridgeline can be
hot and dry in summer. A fresh blanket of snow, though, makes for a rewarding
winter outing on snowshoes. The expanse of hills and low-lying mountains in all
directions is particularly scenic in winter, offering views into Red Butte Canyon
below and the Salt Lake Valley.

Return to the trailhead the way you came. But for your return by car to Salt
Lake City, consider driving down Emigration Canyon. Historical markers along
the way will give you a glimpse into the canyon's early history.

NEARBY ACTIVITIES

Hogle Zoo is at the mouth of Emigration Canyon, across from This Is The Place
Heritage Park. The zoo's animals and exhibits, spread over 42 acres, see more
than 700,000 visitors per year. Open year-round and closed only on Christmas
and New Year's Day; call 801-582-1631 or visit **hoglezoo.org** to learn about special
exhibits and programs.

CITY CREEK CANYON 13

IN BRIEF

With the 26-story LDS Church office building to your back and the Utah state capitol in front of you, follow a creek through a city park, quickly leaving the city behind. Within 2 miles you'll be walking in a national forest and nature preserve shared with elk, moose, and mountain lions.

DESCRIPTION

City Creek has served as Salt Lake City's primary water source since 1847, when Mormon pioneers first arrived in the valley. No other hike in the United States allows you to be in an urban center, within a block of the state capitol, then so quickly find yourself following a tumbling creek through the depths of a protected canyon filled with undisturbed wildlife and dense vegetation.

If the hardest part of this hike is finding parking, then the most dangerous part is crossing the pedestrian crosswalk on State Street to access the "trailhead." Starting at the northeast corner of State Street and North Temple, walk one-half block to the east along the decorative sidewalk and continue as the sidewalk curves north onto Canyon Road, away from downtown and into a quiet residential area. Tiles embedded in the concrete identify native animals and birds by their footprints, preparing you for what you're likely to find up-canyon.

On July 21, 1847, near the location of the trailhead, Orson Pratt and Erastus Snow (along with other members of the vanguard party) arrived in the Salt Lake Valley and set up camp. They quickly diverted water from City Creek to soften the soil. By the time Brigham Young arrived three days later, they had already planted 5 acres of potatoes. Within

KEY AT-A-GLANCE INFORMATION

LENGTH: 2–9 miles

ELEVATION GAIN: 300–740'

ELEVATION: 4,370' (main trailhead), 4,705' (alternate trailhead)

CONFIGURATION: Out-and-back or one-way

DIFFICULTY: Easy

SCENERY: Riparian canyon with brushy slopes; good bird-watching

EXPOSURE: Partially shaded

TRAFFIC: Moderate–heavy

TRAIL SURFACE: Paved or dirt, depending on options chosen

HIKING TIME: 1–4 hours

WATER REQUIREMENTS: 0.5 liter; water fountains along trail

SEASON: Year-round

ACCESS: No fees or permits

MAPS: USGS Salt Lake City North

FACILITIES: Restrooms near trailhead and at several places along the parkway

DOGS: On leash

SPECIAL COMMENTS: City Creek is a multiuse trail, popular with cyclists, joggers, strollers, and hikers. Hikers may choose from dozens of spur trails and dirt trails that parallel the paved parkway.

GPS TRAILHEAD COORDINATES

Main trailhead:
N40° 46.300´ W111° 53.280´
Alternate canyon trailhead:
N40° 47.517´ W111° 53.280´

Directions ➜

It seems strange to refer to one of the busiest intersections in downtown Salt Lake City as a trailhead. Yet the hike starts at the northeast corner of State Street (US 89) and North Temple, just a block from Temple Square and convenient to downtown hotels and shopping. The most difficult part of getting to the trailhead will be finding a place to park. Use one of the public or commercial lots nearby—most street parking in the vicinity is limited to 2 hours.

You can also start the hike farther up the canyon by driving to the City Creek Nature Preserve entrance area. Take North Temple west 0.3 mile to B Street (250 East). Turn left on B Street and continue north 0.7 mile through the Avenues neighborhood. At the corner of B Street and 11th Avenue, B Street becomes East Bonneville Boulevard. Continue north 0.6 mile on East Bonneville Boulevard along the east rim of City Creek Canyon. As East Bonneville Boulevard makes a hairpin turn, go right onto the narrow paved road leading into the City Creek Nature Preserve (marked by a large sign). Drive 0.1 mile to the small parking area at the gateway entrance to City Creek Canyon.

a matter of weeks, a grist mill had been built on City Creek. During the early years of Salt Lake City, energy harnessed from the creek powered many essential industries, such as blacksmith shops, furniture makers, and clothing mills. Water from City Creek still supplies drinking water for much of downtown Salt Lake City and the Avenues.

After walking through two residential blocks, pass through the gate at the entrance of Memory Grove Park. As you enter the park, the rising canyon walls have already blocked the view of the city, and it's easy to forget that the capitol building is just 400 feet to your left but completely out of sight.

Once within the park, walk along the main paved road or on any of the pathways that pass the various monuments and benches placed throughout. Several footbridges cross the creek and allow you to use the dirt trail on the creek's east side. This trail hugs the creek and provides more shade, solitude, and varied terrain than the paved parkway. It normally delivers a sure footing but can be slick during snowmelt or after a heavy rain.

Follow the creek up Memory Grove Park and through a second gate. After 1.5 miles, the paved parkway curves to the right and crosses over City Creek to join Bonneville Boulevard. Take the narrower paved trail that rises to the left, passing the retention pond on your right (often home to ducks and geese). This area provides a convenient turnaround point for a 3-mile round-trip hike, or you can cross Bonneville Boulevard and enter the City Creek Nature Preserve, straight ahead.

After crossing Bonneville Boulevard, walk 0.1 mile to a small parking area with an entrance station, water fountain, and restrooms. You can use this area as an alternate trailhead, allowing you to bypass the hassle of downtown parking and begin your hike in more of a wilderness setting. The road, which continues up the canyon, closes to vehicle traffic October 30–May 25, and even when it's open, cars are allowed only on even-numbered days. The city manages the area beyond the entrance station as a protected watershed and wildlife refuge.

As you walk up the paved parkway, remember that you're sharing the road with cyclists, who often come down the canyon at high speeds. Hikers should stay on the side of the road nearest the creek.

About 800 feet past the entrance station, a trail (marked by a sign) heads up the hillside to the left. This trail, which parallels the creek and the parkway up the canyon, provides a quieter, more natural alternative to the parkway. It follows the gentle slope of the canyon hillside, which is covered by grasses, dense brush, and Gambel oaks. Expect both less shade and less traffic on the trail, which still provides easy access to the frequent restrooms and drinking fountains along the parkway. To the right of the parkway, City Creek descends the canyon in a series of meandering stretches punctuated by dozens of small waterfalls.

The canyon is a year-round home to deer, coyote, and elusive mountain lions. In winter, you may well spot elk and moose, even in the lower elevations below the reservoir. Bird-watchers enjoy the abundant and varied raptor populations throughout the year. Hawks, eagles, falcons, and owls find small rodents on the canyon's grassy slopes to be easy pickings. Grouse, quail, chukar, and pheasants are plentiful in the brush.

Along both the creek and parkway, cottonwoods offer ample shade. About 2 miles from the entrance station, the higher elevation and north-facing slope provide a hospitable environment for stands of balsam and spruce. Scattered along the parkway are convenient rest areas with picnic tables, restrooms, and water fountains, making City Creek Canyon a popular destination for family outings, picnics, and outdoor relaxation.

From the entrance station, City Creek continues up the canyon for 13 miles, and the road is paved for 5.8 miles. The creek is fed by snowmelt, natural springs at the top of the canyon, and many smaller springs along the course of the creek. A reservoir, 3 miles from the entrance station, makes a convenient turnaround point. Because the area is a protected watershed, no dogs are permitted above the reservoir.

Although most visitors to City Creek Canyon stay close to the parkway, creek, and main trail, dozens of side trails lead up the slopes on either side of the canyon. In less than 15 minutes from a creekside picnic area, you can reach the ridge, which offers commanding views of the Salt Lake Valley to the south.

NEARBY ACTIVITIES

Because the hike originates in **downtown Salt Lake City,** shopping malls, restaurants, theaters, and hotels are close by. Historic Temple Square is just a block to the west, and the Utah State Capitol is two blocks to the north. Before starting the hike, you may want to walk through the Brigham Young Historic Park, on the southeast corner of State Street and North Temple. The park features a waterwheel, mill, and other displays depicting the role of City Creek in Salt Lake City history.

RED BUTTE GARDEN

IN BRIEF

Just minutes by foot from the University of Utah campus, formal gardens give way to natural-area trails in a peaceful setting of beauty and historical significance that also provides education and fun. There's something for everyone at any time of year.

DESCRIPTION

It would be easy to visit Red Butte Garden and spend the better part of a day enjoying the colorful floral gardens, ponds, and waterfalls without ever venturing into the more-remote natural area. Indeed, most visitors find sufficient variety and entertainment in the 18 acres of landscaped gardens that they never leave the paved trails for the nearly 100 acres of grassy hillsides, wildflower meadows, and rocky outcrops that lie to the east of the formal gardens. But those who come prepared with basic trail shoes and water can enjoy a network of more than 4 miles of hill trails, offering gentle ascents that lead to sweeping views of the Salt Lake Valley.

Beginning in the late 1800s, the U.S. Army used the strategically important hillside as a camp, firing range, and fort. The red-sandstone crags that form the hill's main ridge served as a quarry that was actively worked

KEY AT-A-GLANCE INFORMATION

LENGTH: 2–4 miles, depending on route and side trails taken

ELEVATION GAIN: 410'

ELEVATION: 5,065' (Courtyard Garden)

CONFIGURATION: Loop with various side trails and extensions

DIFFICULTY: Easy–moderate

SCENERY: Foothills, outcrops of red sandstone, riparian corridor, valley views

EXPOSURE: Full sun, partial shade

TRAFFIC: High in formal gardens, low in natural area

TRAIL SURFACE: Paved in formal gardens, dirt trails in natural area

HIKING TIME: 1–2 hours

WATER REQUIREMENTS: 1 liter

SEASON: Open year-round; hours vary by season.

ACCESS: Entrance fee paid at visitor center (see page 4); garden members admitted free

MAPS: USGS Sugar House

FACILITIES: Restrooms, water, snacks, phone at visitor center

DOGS: Prohibited

Directions

From Salt Lake City, take either I-80 east to Foothill Drive (Exit 129) or I-215 north to Foothill Drive (Exit 1). Continue north 3.1 miles on Foothill Drive (UT 186) to Wakara Way. Turn right on Wakara Way and continue 0.6 mile to the Red Butte Garden entrance. Parking is 0.1 mile ahead on the left. Enter the garden and trail system through the visitor center.

GPS TRAILHEAD COORDINATES

Courtyard Garden:
N40° 45.929´ W111° 49.422´

Red Butte Garden

until about 1934, producing the redstone blocks still seen in many of the prominent homes and buildings throughout the Salt Lake Valley.

At the visitor center you'll receive a useful guide and map that identify many of the garden highlights, such as the Courtyard Garden, the Herb Garden, the Water Pavilion, and the Children's Garden. The guide also features a map of the natural-area trails, showing four different trailheads that access the natural area from the formal gardens.

One popular trail loop follows the perimeter of the Red Butte Garden property and offers a surprising variety of terrain, foliage, and scenery in a 2-mile hike. Beginning at the Courtyard Garden, just outside the visitor center, take the trail for 200 feet along the south side of the Four Seasons Garden. Leaving the formal area, continue to the right along a wide, bark path, cross the Quarry Road, and continue up the Seepy Hollow Trail for 0.2 mile to another Quarry Road crossing. Seepy Hollow follows the course of a natural spring seepage, so in wet conditions you might want to take the longer Quarry Road. A short 0.1-mile walk up Quarry Road brings you to a sign marking the junction of the Zeke's Mountain Trail loop to the left.

From this junction you can take a 0.1-mile spur trail to the end of Quarry Road and visit the historic Quarry House. This fascinating sandstone structure, dating to the late 1800s, was built to store equipment and house the quarry superintendent. Although the roof is gone and some of the walls have been vandalized, the house's stonework shows the masons' enduring craftsmanship. The centerpiece of the Quarry House is a large double-sided fireplace.

Returning to Zeke's Mountain Trail, you'll wind through a thicket of Gambel oak up the craggy hillside to the Bennett Vista Trail, which leads to the hill's crest and offers commanding views of the Salt Lake Valley. From the hilltop, continue east on Zeke's Mountain Trail, generally following the property's fenced perimeter. At the far east side of the property, the trail meets the fence. Here, a one-way gate allows unwelcome deer to leave the property so they can forage on the adjoining National Forest Service land rather than eat the cultivated flowers in Red Butte Garden.

The trail descends along the fence line to the creek, which forms the northern boundary of the garden. Along the Creekside Trail you'll enjoy the shade of oaks and bigtooth maples. Continue on this trail 0.4 mile before returning to the formal gardens.

Throughout the natural-area trails, you'll find more than 130 native plants and trees. In spring, when the garden is especially colorful, yellow blooms of arrowleaf-balsam root and speckles of blue Wasatch penstemon dot the green hillside. You might see a Great Basin rattlesnake sunning itself on the trail or spot rodents, rabbits, or even evidence of an occasional bobcat.

Red Butte Garden's natural-area trails are well marked with signs at all trailheads. While the signs become more scarce in the outlying areas, getting lost is never much of a concern—the property is fenced on all sides and you can visually

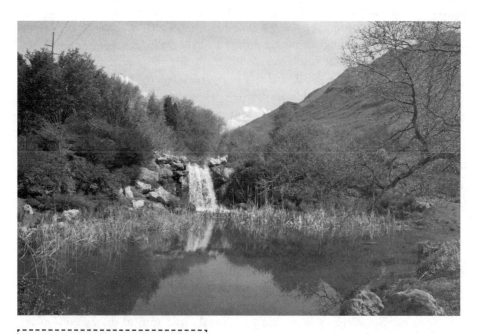

Waterfall and pond at Red Butte Garden

orient yourself along most of the trails. If you're ever in doubt, just follow any trail downhill and to the west, and you'll soon find yourself back within the formal gardens.

The natural-area trails offer plenty of options in the way of short loops, spurs, and side trails. After exploring the foothills and creekside in the natural area, you can return to the wide, paved trails of the formal gardens and easily spend an additional hour or more enjoying the year-round beauty in this community treasure.

NEARBY ACTIVITIES

Red Butte Garden (300 Wakara Way) offers a year-round program of classes, workshops, activities, tours, and community programs. The Outdoor Concert Series features world-renowned performing artists on the garden's amphitheater stage during June, July, and August. Call 801-585-0556 or visit **redbuttegarden.org** for a schedule and tickets. The garden lies adjacent to the University of Utah, which provides an abundant offering of concerts, sporting events, and campus activities.

THE LIVING ROOM
(with Red Butte Extension) 15

IN BRIEF

The Living Room is the best room in the house for an accessible overview of the Salt Lake Valley. It's furnished with charming sandstone chairs, armrests, and even coffee tables you can put your feet on. The hike leads through foothill vegetation and offers an onward scramble to a higher sandstone outcrop on a ridge above Red Butte Canyon.

DESCRIPTION

Red Butte Canyon is the smallest of seven canyons streaming down the Wasatch ridges east of Salt Lake City. It lies directly east of downtown Salt Lake City and above Fort Douglas and the University of Utah campus. A hike to the popular Living Room overlook will take you through foothill vegetation to Red Butte Ridge, which forms the south side of Red Butte Canyon.

The historical significance of the area was first tied to its use as a sandstone quarry and later to water rights. In 1862, U.S. troops established Fort Douglas and used the spring water of Red Butte Creek for domestic and irrigation purposes, affecting the 3,000 local residents who relied on the creek for their water supply. Today the canyon is managed as

KEY AT-A-GLANCE INFORMATION

LENGTH: 2.3 miles round-trip to Living Room, 2.7 miles round-trip to Red Butte extension

ELEVATION GAIN: 980' to Living Room + 360' to Red Butte extension

ELEVATION AT TRAILHEAD: 5,000'

CONFIGURATION: Out-and-back

DIFFICULTY: Easy

SCENERY: Foothills, valley views

EXPOSURE: Partial shade to Living Room, unshaded from Living Room to Red Butte extension

TRAFFIC: Moderate

TRAIL SURFACE: Dirt and gravel to Living Room, rock to Red Butte extension

HIKING TIME: 1.5–2 hours round-trip to Living Room; 2–3 hours round-trip to Red Butte extension

WATER REQUIREMENTS: 1 liter

SEASON: Spring, summer, fall

ACCESS: No fees or permits

MAPS: USGS Fort Douglas

FACILITIES: No restrooms or water at trailhead

DOGS: Permitted (waste must be bagged and removed)

SPECIAL COMMENTS: A popular sunset hike for locals

Directions

From Salt Lake City take either I-80 east to Foothill Drive (Exit 129) or I-215 north to Foothill Drive (Exit 1). Continue north 3.1 miles on Foothill Drive (UT 186) to Wakara Way. Turn right on Wakara Way and continue 0.6 mile to the Red Butte Garden entrance. Turn right on Colorow Drive before entering Red Butte Garden, and continue 0.2 mile to the trailhead, on the left side of the street.

GPS TRAILHEAD COORDINATES

N40° 45.557´ W111° 49.277´

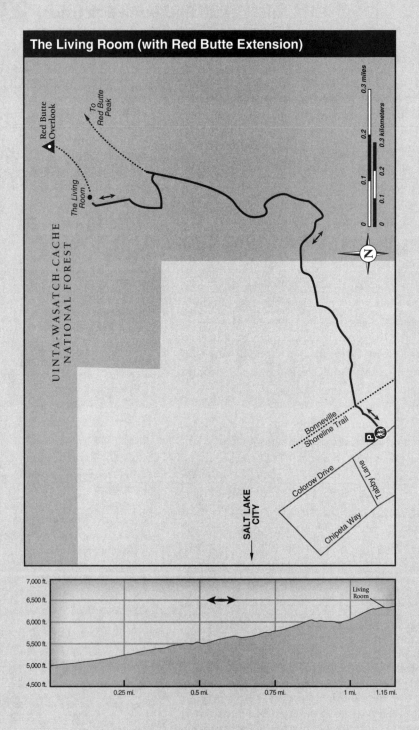

The Living Room (with Red Butte Extension)

Russian olive tree near trail

a protected Natural Research Area under the control of the U.S. Forest Service and is recognized as the most pristine watershed along the Wasatch Front.

Within 100 yards of the marked trailhead on the east side of Colorow Drive, you come to a small spring-fed creek. The trail crosses the creek at the base of a large, mature Russian olive tree, one of several in the riparian corridor. The path continues up the slope for another 0.1 mile before arriving at the wide Bonneville Shoreline Trail. Here you take a jog to the right for 50 feet before continuing up and to the left along a gravel trail. You'll enter a dense cover of Gambel oak and bigtooth maple near the mouth of a small ravine known as Georges Hollow.

At 0.7 mile from the trailhead, the route breaks out onto a ridgeline that you'll follow up and to the east along the south slope of a ravine. At 1.1 miles, you come to a trail junction at the top of the ravine. Continuing straight ahead leads up to the 6,472-foot Red Butte peak. Instead, take the trail that crosses the ravine and curves to the left. This path to the Living Room now makes a westward ascent along the north side of the ravine. Upon crossing to the north side of the ravine, the rocks change from gray limestone to peach-colored sandstone. After walking just 0.1 mile from the junction along the sandstone-studded slope, you arrive at the Living Room.

The Living Room invites a relaxing stay. A man-made arrangement of angular sandstone slabs provides a comfortable observation point complete with several chairs, armrests, ottomans, and coffee tables. There's no better place to sit

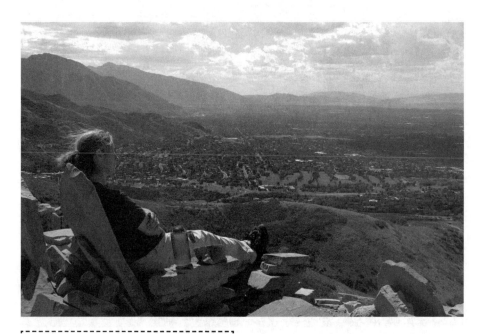

Stone lounge chairs await at the Living Room.

and watch a sunset, take in the spring wildflowers or fall colors, or just relax and enjoy a snack. The Living Room overlooks the University of Utah and Fort Douglas, where athletes were housed during the 2002 Winter Olympics. The extended views stretch from the Great Salt Lake to the north to the Oquirrh Mountains in the west, and down to the southern end of the Salt Lake Valley, clear to the Point of the Mountain.

While the Living Room is the final destination for most hikers, you can undertake an easy scramble to a higher overlook if you have a little extra energy. Behind the Living Room, a faint and noticeably steeper trail leads up the sandstone crags to the east along a ridgeline to a clearly visible viewpoint. In about 15 minutes, you'll find yourself on a shelf of large sandstone slabs with views down into Red Butte Canyon and the Red Butte Reservoir to the north. The extension to this overlook adds about 0.4 mile round-trip beyond the Living Room.

NEARBY ACTIVITIES

Ensign Peak is a popular Salt Lake overlook with a well-maintained trail and a round-trip distance of less than 1 mile. From downtown, take State Street to the east of the State Capitol Building on East Capitol Boulevard. Continue up to Edgecombe Drive, turn left, and continue 0.4 mile to the trailhead, on the left at Ensign Peak Nature Park.

SUMMIT PARK PEAK 16

IN BRIEF

This is a real rarity in the Wasatch—a trail that's as enjoyable for mountain bikers as it is for hikers and snowshoers. The peak, which straddles the Summit–Salt Lake county line, affords great views in all directions.

DESCRIPTION

As the trail rises from the roadside trailhead, you might wonder why the gradient is so much gentler than those of other Wasatch trails, which typically start steep and get steeper. The reason—this is a purpose-built mountain bike trail. The sculpted contour, wide turns, smooth surface, and mild incline were custom-made for mountain bikers. The trail was also expertly crafted to be sustainable and erosion-resistant. Even though this is a shared trail, there's plenty of room and good visibility, so it's safe and fun for both hikers and bikers.

The initial ten switchbacks on the signed Short Stack Trail lead through a forest of mature white fir, spruce, and quaking aspen. At 1.1 miles the dense forest cover opens to views to the east, and in another 0.2 mile you'll follow

KEY AT-A-GLANCE INFORMATION

LENGTH: 6 miles round-trip
ELEVATION GAIN: 1,250'
ELEVATION AT TRAILHEAD: 7,368'
CONFIGURATION: Out-and-back or balloon
DIFFICULTY: Moderate
SCENERY: Canyon, ridgeline, and mountain views
EXPOSURE: Almost entirely shaded
TRAFFIC: Moderate
TRAIL SURFACE: Dirt, rock
HIKING TIME: 2.5–3.5 hours
WATER REQUIREMENTS: 1–2 liters
SEASON: Late spring, summer, fall; snowshoeing in winter
ACCESS: No fees or permits. Summit Park Trails are managed by the Snyderville Basin Recreation District of Summit County.
MAPS: USGS Park City West
FACILITIES: No restrooms or water at trailhead
DOGS: On leash

Directions ⟶

Take I-80 east of Salt Lake City to the Parleys Summit turnoff (Exit 140). At the end of the off-ramp, turn right and take another immediate right onto Aspen Drive. Continue west on Aspen Drive up the hill. In 0.5 mile the street veers left and changes to Crestview Drive. Continue another 0.5 mile, and the street name changes again to Innsbruck Strasse. In another 0.5 mile, at the end of the paved street, take the dirt road to your right another 100 yards as it curves to the left. The signed trailhead is on your right, past the curve. Park on the side of the dirt road.

GPS TRAILHEAD COORDINATES

N40° 44.553´ W111° 37.078´

Summit Park Peak

Summit Park trails are popular with bikers and hikers.

the signed Road to WOS, where the trail will occasionally open to views into Toll Canyon to the east. (There seems to be some local mystery regarding who or what WOS is. The answer is simple: it's an acronym for "Weather Observation Station.")

At 1.5 miles from the trailhead you'll come to a trail junction. Again, stay on the clearly marked Road to WOS until you arrive at a ridgetop clearing and trail junction, 2.4 miles from your starting trailhead.

Take the Over Easy Trail to your right. This is where the mountain bikers part company with the hikers. The trail steepens, narrows, and quickly becomes faint in places. Continue upward on this trail as it rises onto a limestone outcropping. Within another 100 yards, you'll be on the summit (also the county line) and be rewarded with fine views. To the east, you'll gaze into Park City and the Snyderville Basin; to the west, you'll look down into Lambs Canyon and enjoy distant views into the Wasatch.

You'll see what look like hiking trails leading down to Lambs Canyon, but don't be tempted to take them unless you want to spend the rest of the day hopelessly bushwhacking. They're actually game trails that never reliably connect with Lambs Canyon. Instead, descend about 100 yards to the base of the summit on the same trail you used for your ascent.

At the base of the summit, in the small clearing, you have the option of turning right and returning on the same trail. But for some variety, and with no more distance, you can continue north on the Over Easy Trail as it undulates along the wide ridge, passes an old lean-to shelter, and eventually drops back down to connect with the Road to WOS at the Grease Mark Trail junction, where you can turn left and make your return to the Short Stack Trail. This return is unmarked and unmaintained, as are the lower trails, but it makes for an enjoyable loop and gives you a longer stay on the upper ridge.

NEARBY ACTIVITIES

The popular **Tanger Outlets** complex in Park City comprises more than 60 brand-name stores, including such outdoors-oriented ones as Eddie Bauer and Columbia Sportswear. To get there, continue east on I-80 another 5 miles to Exit 145. Before you go, check for discounts at **tangeroutlet.com/parkcity/coupons.**

LAMBS CANYON 17

IN BRIEF

Old-growth forests of spruce and fir, shared with quaking aspen, line a canyon fed by several springs. A steep trail to an 8,100-foot pass offers views into the valley before leading down Elbow Fork and into Mill Creek Canyon. It's a symphony of woods, wildflowers, berries, creeks, and views. This is a great snowshoe trail in the depths of winter, and easily accessed on cross-country skis along Mill Creek Canyon.

DESCRIPTION

In the 1860s, Abel Lamb recognized the value of the timber in the canyon that now bears his name. He built a cabin in the canyon, and his son, Horace, built a sawmill. To meet the construction demands in the growing Salt Lake Valley, the sawmill hauled lumber down the new Golden Pass Toll Road (now I-80), which

----

Directions

LAMBS CANYON TRAILHEAD: Take I-80 east from Salt Lake City to Lambs Canyon (Exit 137). Turn right onto Lambs Canyon Road and drive 2 miles up the canyon to the trailhead parking area, on the left. The trailhead is across the street, on the west side of Lambs Canyon Road.

ELBOW FORK TRAILHEAD (MILL CREEK CANYON): From I-215 on Salt Lake City's east side, take the 3300 South/3900 South turnoff (Exit 4). Turn left onto Wasatch Boulevard and go north 1 block to 3800 South. Turn right on 3800 South and continue toward the mouth of Mill Creek Canyon. Pass the toll booth at 0.7 mile and continue another 5.3 miles to the Elbow Fork trailhead, where Mill Creek and the road turn sharply to the right. Roadside parking is available at the trailhead.

KEY AT-A-GLANCE INFORMATION

LENGTH: 4 miles one-way

ELEVATION GAIN: 1,518'

ELEVATION: 6,615' (Lambs Canyon), 6,686' (Elbow Fork)

CONFIGURATION: Out-and-back or one-way

DIFFICULTY: Moderate

SCENERY: Abundant plant life in two deep canyons, views of Salt Lake Valley and surrounding peaks from pass

EXPOSURE: Mostly shaded

TRAFFIC: Light

TRAIL SURFACE: Dirt

HIKING TIME: 2.5–3.5 hours

WATER REQUIREMENTS: 1–2 liters; water in creeks can be purified.

SEASON: Year-round

ACCESS: Mill Creek Canyon is a fee-access area within Uinta-Wasatch-Cache National Forest (see page 4). The Maple Grove gate is closed November 1–July 1. To hike Lambs Canyon when the gate is closed, park at the Maple Grove picnic area and walk 1.5 miles up the canyon road to the Elbow Fork trailhead.

MAPS: USGS Mount Aire, Trails Illustrated Wasatch Front (709)

FACILITIES: Vault toilets at trailheads

DOGS: Prohibited in Lambs Canyon

GPS TRAILHEAD COORDINATES

Lambs Canyon:
N40° 43.277´ W111° 39.490´
Elbow Fork:
N40° 42.397´ W111° 41.408´

Lambs Canyon

Lambs Canyon

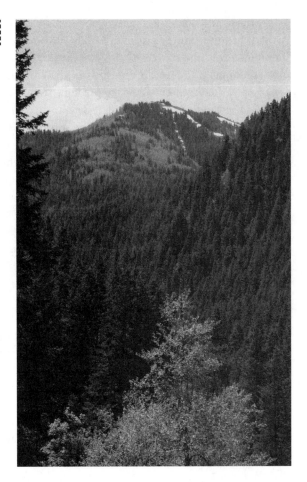

was constructed by Parley P. Pratt through Big Canyon (now known as Parleys Canyon). But Lamb's sawmill couldn't make a dent in the thousands of acres of timber that still covers Lambs Canyon today.

You can explore Lambs Canyon in a variety of ways, and the one-way canyon-to-canyon route described here requires a shuttle vehicle left at either end. The hike leads from Lambs Canyon to Mill Creek Canyon via the Great Western Trail and Elbow Fork. You can just as easily undertake this hike as a 4-mile out-and-back within Lambs Canyon. Just park at the Lambs Canyon trailhead, hike to the pass for views into the valley, and then return back down the trail to your car. This out-and-back Lambs Canyon option also avoids the access fee for Mill Creek Canyon.

The Lambs Canyon Trail also serves as a section of the Great Western Trail, which, when completed, will stretch continuously from Mexico to Canada and traverse some of the most spectacular scenery in the West. The Lambs Canyon section, from I-80 to Mill Creek, is one of the most beautifully wooded and shaded sections of the trail.

From the Lambs Canyon trailhead parking area, cross Lambs Canyon Road and immediately cross a bridge over a stream lined with willows. Immediately, you're engulfed in a forest of aspen, fir, and spruce—but don't ignore the foliage at your feet. Wild strawberries, raspberries, grapes, and mint line the trail. In spring, mulesear, wyethia, larkspur, and harebell brighten the trail—and as long as they're not on your lawn, even dandelions are a welcome wildflower in the woods. Diverse shrubbery also lines the narrow trail and makes long pants preferable. The soil is dark and well packed, sprinkled with fir needles and ribboned with roots of trees.

Moose and deer find Lambs Canyon a welcoming habitat. Watch for the burrows of ground squirrels near the trail, and look out for wrens, varied thrushes, hummingbirds, and sparrows.

At about 1.5 miles up the canyon, the trail departs the spring and enters a series of wide, steep switchbacks through stands of aspen as you approach the pass. At the saddle elevation of 8,133 feet, the woods open up to views of Gobblers Knob and Mount Raymond to the south and Grandeur Peak to the west. To the left of Grandeur Peak, you can also see a slice of the Salt Lake Valley.

From the saddle at the top of the pass, you have a choice based on where your car is waiting. You can return to Lambs Canyon for an out-and-back hike or continue on down Elbow Fork into Mill Creek Canyon for a one-way hike with all-new territory.

The trail from the pass down to Mill Creek is slightly less shaded than the trail leading up from Lambs Canyon. Still, within minutes you drop into the canyon along a gathering creek and soon find yourself back in the shade. The trail through Elbow Fork lacks the diversity of foliage found in Lambs Canyon but offers some fine views of the surrounding canyon and occasional glimpses of the sandstone crags on Mount Aire to the north.

At 1.8 miles from the pass, and less than 0.2 mile from the Elbow Fork trailhead, you come to a trail junction. The fork to the right leads up the main branch of Elbow Fork on the Mount Aire Trail. Take the fork to the left to return to the Elbow Fork trailhead and Mill Creek Canyon Road. Remember that the gate to the upper canyon, at Maple Grove, is open only from July 1 to November 1. If you want to access Elbow Fork outside of that season, you'll need to park at Maple Grove and hike an additional 1.5 miles to the trailhead. But a shaded walk on a car-free road with Mill Creek at your side can be enchanting.

NEARBY ACTIVITIES

The **Mill Creek Canyon Fishing Dock and Boardwalk** is at the Terraces, just 4.4 miles up the canyon on the right-hand side of the road. A short 0.1-mile walk leads to fishing fun for young and old.

MOUNT AIRE 18

IN BRIEF

Tucked away on the ridge behind Grandeur Peak, Mount Aire is not visible from most of Salt Lake City. Still, it offers excellent views to the east and of surrounding peaks. The Mount Aire Trail connects with many other Mill Creek trails and the Great Western Trail.

DESCRIPTION

Mount Aire is a bite-sized challenge. If you're in great shape, you can drive to the trailhead after work, bag the summit, and be back to your car in 2.5 hours. If you're looking to build speed and endurance, Mount Aire offers a steep and steady incline for nearly 2 miles that will let you know if you're ready for a more demanding adventure. It's also an ideal snowshoe ascent in winter that offers a real challenge, rewarding you with great views of snow-covered peaks and hills in all directions.

During the summer you can drive directly to the Elbow Fork Trailhead and go straight to the summit in just 1.9 miles. From November 1 to July 1 (with some variation based on weather), the gate at Maple Grove is closed to motor vehicles, so you'll have to walk or ski the 1.5 miles from Maple Grove up to the Elbow Fork Trailhead. Walking along the shaded road

KEY AT-A-GLANCE INFORMATION

LENGTH: 3.8 miles round-trip

ELEVATION GAIN: 1,987'

ELEVATION AT TRAILHEAD: 6,686'

CONFIGURATION: Out-and-back

DIFFICULTY: Moderate

SCENERY: Wooded canyon leading to a summit with panoramic views

EXPOSURE: Mostly shaded the first mile up to ridgeline saddle; partially shaded to summit

TRAFFIC: Light

TRAIL SURFACE: Dirt, rock

HIKING TIME: 2.5–4 hours

WATER REQUIREMENTS: 1–2 liters

SEASON: Year-round

ACCESS: Mill Creek Canyon is a fee-access area within Uinta-Wasatch-Cache National Forest (see page 4). The Maple Grove gate is closed November 1–July 1. To hike Mount Aire when the gate is closed, park at the Maple Grove picnic area and walk 1.5 miles up the canyon road to the Elbow Fork Trailhead.

MAPS: USGS Mount Aire, Trails Illustrated Wasatch Front (709)

FACILITIES: Vault toilet at trailhead. No drinking water at trailhead. Water in creek should be purified.

DOGS: Must be leashed on even-numbered days; can be unleashed on odd-numbered days

---

Directions

From I-215 on Salt Lake City's east side, take the 3300 South/3900 South turnoff (Exit 4). Turn left onto Wasatch Boulevard and go north 1 block to 3800 South. Turn right on 3800 South and continue toward the mouth of Mill Creek Canyon. Pass the toll booth at 0.7 mile and continue another 5.3 miles to the Elbow Fork Trailhead, where Mill Creek and the road turn sharply to the right. Roadside parking is available at the trailhead.

GPS TRAILHEAD COORDINATES

N40° 42.397´ W111° 41.408´

Mount Aire

Gobblers Knob from Mount Aire

as it follows Mill Creek up the canyon is really quite enjoyable, even if it adds 3 miles to the round-trip.

The Elbow Fork trailhead lies at the point where Mill Creek and the road make a sharp 90-degree turn to the south. The trailhead also provides access to the Lambs Canyon Trail, the Pipeline Trail, and the Great Western Trail. Within 0.1 mile of the trailhead, you come to a well-marked fork in the trail, with the Mount Aire Trail taking off to the left. It quickly crosses a footbridge over the small creek and follows the creek up a deep, shaded canyon filled with Douglas-fir, maple, and quaking aspen at the higher elevations.

Continue following the trail along the Elbow Fork tributary for 0.8 mile to the point where the creek is just a trickle. At that point the trail ascends a series of short, steep switchbacks, and within less than a minute you're high above the creek on the east slope of the side canyon. Within another 0.2 mile you emerge from the canyon's shade to arrive at the ridgeline saddle, which offers views down Parleys Canyon to the north. A faint, unmaintained trail follows the ridgeline to the west. With some advance planning you could take this trail to Grandeur Peak and descend to Mill Creek through Church Fork. But for now, keep to the right and set your sights on Mount Aire to the east.

Leaving the saddle, the trail winds through the sandstone along Mount Aire's western and southern slopes. This sandstone formation, while unusual for the Wasatch, is the same formation you see on Grandeur Peak and along the entire ridge. Although the climb along the upper slope is largely shadeless, it is scented with sage and arrowleaf-balsam root. While the trail is easy to follow during most of the year, adding a foot or more of snow in the winter could pose some route-finding challenges.

Nearing the summit, you come to an overlook with impressive views of the densely wooded slopes of upper Mill Creek Canyon and Gobblers Knob to the south. From this overlook, a sharp turn to the north leads to the summit just 100 yards ahead. Although the summit ridge extends to the north for more than 200 yards, the true summit is the rocky sandstone outcrop first reached from the south. From this spot you can frequently watch eagles soaring high above the canyon. Below and to the east, you'll see I-80 leading toward Park City. The Salt Lake Valley views to the west are limited, but the panoramic views of mountains in all directions go on forever.

NEARBY ACTIVITIES

Most visitors to **Mill Creek Canyon** find so much to keep them busy—picnicking, hiking, bicycling, mountain biking, snowshoeing, and skiing—that they never seem to have much need for add-ons. But if you have an extra 30 minutes at the end of your hike, consider driving another 3.5 miles up to the top of the canyon to scout your next adventure. When the pavement ends at the Big Water trailhead, you're at an elevation of more than 8,000 feet. From this point you can access the Great Western Trail, or the Desolation Trail into Big Cottonwood Canyon, opening the door to hundreds of miles of hiking and biking trails.

GRANDEUR PEAK 19

IN BRIEF

Grandeur Peak delivers a lot of bang for the buck. One of the most easily accessible peaks along the Wasatch Front, it offers both great trail conditions and commanding views in all directions.

DESCRIPTION

Imagine a warm Saturday in spring. Snow still flanks most of the high peaks surrounding Salt Lake City. You pull out your hiking boots and decide to bag a mountain summit—something impressive, something grand. Grandeur Peak is the perfect pursuit. It lies at the forefront of the ridge just north of Mount Olympus and to the south of Parleys Canyon and I-80. It may not be as high as Mount Timpanogos or Pfeifferhorn, or as instantly recognizable to local residents as Mount Olympus, but from nearly anywhere in Salt Lake City you can be at the trailhead in 20 minutes and on your way to a mountain adventure.

Mill Creek Canyon is Salt Lake City's favorite picnic destination, and Church Fork is the first picnic site you come to driving up the canyon. If you see cars parked along the canyon road, you can safely assume that the eight

KEY AT-A-GLANCE INFORMATION

LENGTH: 5.4 miles round-trip

ELEVATION GAIN: 2,387'

ELEVATION AT TRAILHEAD: 5,912'

CONFIGURATION: Out-and-back

DIFFICULTY: Moderate

SCENERY: Canyon, mountain, and city views. Trail follows creek up a wooded side canyon.

EXPOSURE: Mostly shaded for first mile, mostly exposed for last 1.7 miles to summit

TRAFFIC: Busy

TRAIL SURFACE: Dirt, rock

HIKING TIME: 2.5–4 hours

WATER REQUIREMENTS: 1–2 liters

SEASON: Spring, summer, fall

ACCESS: Mill Creek Canyon is a fee-access area within Uinta-Wasatch-Cache National Forest (see page 4). From the trailhead to the switchbacks, you will be crossing property owned by the Boy Scouts of America.

MAPS: USGS Mt. Aire, Sugar House, Trails Illustrated Wasatch Front (709)

FACILITIES: Restrooms and water at trailhead

DOGS: Must be leashed on even-numbered days; can be unleashed on odd-numbered days

---

Directions

From I-215 on Salt Lake City's east side, take the 3300 South/3900 South turnoff (Exit 4). Turn left onto Wasatch Boulevard and go north 1 block to 3800 South. Turn right on 3800 South and continue toward the mouth of Mill Creek Canyon. Pass the toll booth at 0.7 mile and continue another 2.3 miles to the Church Fork Picnic area, on your left. If the gate is open, turn left and drive 0.3 mile up through the picnic area to a small trailhead parking area at the end of the road.

GPS TRAILHEAD COORDINATES

N40° 42.038´ W111° 44.552´

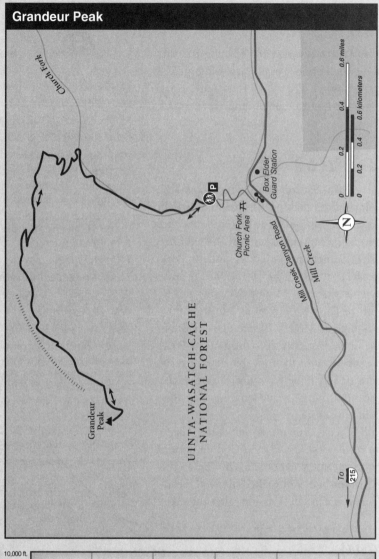

Grandeur Peak

Church Fork

Box Elder
Guard Station

P

Church Fork
Picnic Area

Mill Creek Canyon Road

Mill Creek

UINTA-WASATCH-CACHE
NATIONAL FOREST

Grandeur
Peak

To 215

N

0.6 miles

0.4

0.6 kilometers

0.2

0.4

0

0.2

0

10,000 ft.					
9,000 ft.					Grandeur Peak
8,000 ft.					
7,000 ft.					
6,000 ft.	Church Fork				
5,000 ft.					

0.5 mi.　　1 mi.　　1.5 mi.　　2 mi.　　2.5 mi.　2.8 mi.

Ridgeline approach to Grandeur Peak

parking spaces at the trailhead are already filled. You might as well park on the shoulder of Mill Creek Canyon Road and walk through the Church Fork picnic area to the trailhead, which is marked by a sign pointing to Grandeur Peak.

Church Fork is a small side canyon on the north side of Mill Creek. It was originally a placer-mining claim that extended from just above the trailhead to near the ridgeline. This claim was deeded to the Boy Scouts of America in 1918 and remains publicly accessible property owned by the Scouts.

After just 0.1 mile on the trail, you'll cross the Pipeline Trail and take a jog to the left, then continue up the canyon on the Grandeur Peak Trail to the right. The trail leads up a steep canyon shaded by maple conifers and bigtooth maples, with Church Fork Creek descending speedily on your right. Along the creekside, the trail is fragrant with fir, wildflowers, wild mint, and arrowleaf-balsam root.

At 0.8 mile, the path begins a series of switchbacks. As you climb the slope, you emerge from the shaded canopy of maple, oak, and fir. From this point on, the trail is largely unshaded. These switchbacks lead toward a sandstone outcrop on the ridge to the north. Below this outcrop, the trail is dotted and bedded with sandstone, uncharacteristic of most Wasatch trails.

As the switchbacks lead up toward the west, you'll have a beautiful straight-on view of Grandeur Peak in front of you, its slopes ribboned with strands of aspen and white fir. At the top of the switchbacks, you'll look to the west and see the

Grandeur Peak viewed from the east

entire trail as it leads to the summit. From this point on, the ascent is steady but more gradual as it follows a route just below the ridgeline through a low covering of Gambel oak.

On your route to the top, you'll come to a crest dotted with juniper. After you've passed this false summit, the true summit lies just 0.2 mile straight ahead. You may see a few patches of snow through late May and sometimes into June along the higher trail. Because hikers, dogs, and bikers share busy Mill Creek Canyon, wildlife sightings are less likely, but you may see deer grazing near the summit in spring and fall.

At 8,299 feet in elevation, the Grandeur Peak summit offers great views in all directions. The Salt Lake Valley spreads out below to the west, and Mount Olympus lies at the front of the next ridge to the south. Behind you, to the northeast, are Mountain Dell and Little Dell reservoirs. Soak up the panoramic views, then enjoy a carefree and relaxing descent.

NEARBY ACTIVITIES

Just a few blocks from the mouth of Mill Creek Canyon, you'll find **REI** (3285 E. 3300 South; 801-486-2100; **rei.com/stores/19**). In addition to selling outdoor gear and offering classes, it's home to the Salt Lake area's Public Lands Information Center, an excellent source of assistance and information about area recreational opportunities.

DESOLATION TRAIL TO SALT LAKE OVERLOOK

20

IN BRIEF

Hiking through a dense forest scented with spruce and fir is just one of the many delights on the Desolation Trail. Climbing over fallen trees and rocky outcrops leads to a direct view of Salt Lake with peaks rising to the north and south.

DESCRIPTION

Don't let the name *Desolation Trail* conjure up images of a dusty, sun-parched ordeal in the desert. Picture a verdant trail cut along a densely wooded hillside with a bed of needles and cones from the various conifers in the canyon.

You'll find the trailhead at the west end of the small South Box Elder parking area. At 0.1 mile, you come to a fork with the Thayne Canyon Trail leading to the left and the Desolation Trail ascending the hillside to the right. To reach the Salt Lake Overlook, stay to the right, although you also have the extended option of a Thayne Canyon–Desolation Trail loop.

The trail navigates a steady series of masterfully crafted and well-groomed switchbacks that reduce the grade on an otherwise precipitous hillside. These northeast slopes provide a cooler, more moist habitat for mosses and a variety of mountain shrubs. In addition to fir and spruce, you'll see maple, Gambel oaks, and

Directions

From I-215 on Salt Lake City's east side, take the 3300 South/3900 South turnoff (Exit 4). Turn left onto Wasatch Boulevard and go north 1 block to 3800 South. Turn right on 3800 South and continue toward the mouth of Mill Creek Canyon. Pass the toll booth at 0.7 mile and continue another 2.5 miles to the South Box Elder trailhead parking area, on the right. A road sign also identifies Desolation Trail 019.

KEY AT-A-GLANCE INFORMATION

LENGTH: 4.8 miles round-trip

ELEVATION GAIN: 1,239'

ELEVATION AT TRAILHEAD: 5,785'

CONFIGURATION: Out-and-back

DIFFICULTY: Moderate

SCENERY: Wooded canyon, city overview

EXPOSURE: Mostly shaded

TRAFFIC: Moderate

TRAIL SURFACE: Dirt, rock

HIKING TIME: 1.5–3 hours

WATER REQUIREMENTS: 1–1.5 liters; no water along trail

SEASON: Spring, summer, fall

ACCESS: Mill Creek Canyon is a fee-access area within Uinta-Wasatch-Cache National Forest (see page 4). From the trailhead to the Salt Lake Overlook, you will be crossing property owned by the Boy Scouts of America. Bicycles are prohibited on the Desolation Trail.

MAPS: USGS Mount Aire, Trails Illustrated Wasatch Front (709)

FACILITIES: Restrooms and water at trailhead

DOGS: Must be leashed on even-numbered days; can be unleashed on odd-numbered days

SPECIAL COMMENTS: This trail, cut along a steep hillside, is particularly susceptible to erosion. Do not shortcut the trails.

GPS TRAILHEAD COORDINATES

N40° 41.850´ W111° 44.400´

Desolation Trail to Salt Lake Overlook

UINTA-WASATCH-CACHE
NATIONAL FOREST

Mill Creek Canyon Road

SALT LAKE
CITY
215

THAYNE CANYON

MOUNT
OLYMPUS
WILDERNESS

Salt Lake
Overlook

N

0   0.1   0.2   0.3 miles

0   0.1   0.2   0.3 kilometers

Canyon and valley views from the overlook

wildflowers along the trail at all elevations. Many fallen trees cross the trail, while others lay parallel to the trail, placed there to fortify the slope against erosion.

At 0.6 mile the trail opens up to sunlight with a patch of Gambel oak, although for most of the hike towering conifers shade hikers. At 0.8 mile the path divides at a rock outcrop. Take the trail on your right, up through the rocky crag.

If you're hiking with young children, be careful of the steep, unprotected drop-offs in many areas where the trail is only a few feet wide. Also, since you're likely to be paying close attention to your feet and the narrow trail, you might well be surprised by a runner or dog coming in the opposite direction. Unleashed dogs appear along the trail frequently on odd-numbered days.

You'll often spot deer and squirrels, and the variety of birds makes Mill Creek Canyon a popular birding destination. Early mornings in summer provide good opportunities to spot blue grouse, Steller's jays, scrub jays, and golden eagles.

At 1.3 miles, a clearing in the woods opens to some beautiful views up Mill Creek Canyon to the east. But the favorite view comes almost by surprise as the trail circles to the west side of the slope. As the trees clear, you'll have a view looking down the canyon with Salt Lake City below. To the north is Grandeur Peak, with Mount Olympus and Hobbs Peak to the south. Several large clusters of jagged rocks offer a place to relax, enjoy the view, and have a snack before heading back down the trail.

Ridgeline views to the south

NEARBY ACTIVITIES

Mill Creek Canyon is Salt Lake City's favorite summer picnic destination. With nine picnic areas within 3–7 miles of the canyon entrance, Mill Creek is the place to go for a weekend brunch or a summer afternoon lunch. Individual sites abound, and group sites accommodate up to 100 people. Many also visit the area for mountain biking, but bikes are allowed on the upper trails only on even-numbered days.

GOBBLERS KNOB
(via Alexander Basin)

IN BRIEF

This popular summit offers great views in all directions, but the most memorable sight will be of the wildflowers that fill Alexander Basin in spring and summer. The steep hike offers some easy scrambling and route-finding up a glacial cirque to the ridge, followed by a short jaunt to the summit.

DESCRIPTION

Although the trail leading to Alexander Basin passes through the Mount Olympus Wilderness, the basin itself is not included in the designated wilderness area. Gobblers Knob is a popular summit climb and Mill Creek is a busy canyon, but Alexander Basin can feel surprisingly remote, even on a summer weekend. Of the four most frequently used trails used to reach the Gobblers Knob summit, Alexander Basin's is the shortest and steepest.

As you drive up Mill Creek Canyon, and especially past the Elbow Fork area, the road narrows and trees on both sides close in to create a sense of being wrapped up in the woods. From the trailhead parking area, you step onto the trail. Within a few seconds, the road disappears and you're engulfed in woods of Douglas-fir and white fir.

Directions ⟶

From I-215 on Salt Lake City's east side, take the 3300 South/3900 South turnoff (Exit 4). Turn left onto Wasatch Boulevard and go north 1 block to 3800 South. Turn right on 3800 South and continue toward the mouth of Mill Creek Canyon. Pass the toll booth at 0.7 mile and continue another 7 miles to the Alexander Basin trailhead (#010). Trailhead parking is on the south side of the road.

ⓘ KEY AT-A-GLANCE INFORMATION

LENGTH: 4.4 miles round-trip

ELEVATION GAIN: 3,106'

ELEVATION AT TRAILHEAD: 7,140'

CONFIGURATION: Out-and-back

DIFFICULTY: Moderate

SCENERY: Wildflowers, alpine basin, summit views

EXPOSURE: Mostly shaded

TRAFFIC: Moderate

TRAIL SURFACE: Dirt to the upper bowl, then rocky to the summit

HIKING TIME: 4–5 hours

SEASON: Summer–early fall. Maple Grove gate to upper Mill Creek Canyon is closed November 1–July 1.

WATER REQUIREMENTS: 2 liters; no perennial water flow near trail

ACCESS: Mill Creek Canyon is a fee-access area within Uinta-Wasatch-Cache National Forest (see page 4).

MAPS: USGS Mount Aire, Trails Illustrated Wasatch Front (709)

FACILITIES: No drinking water or restrooms at trailhead; water in creek should be purified. Restrooms are 1.5 miles from trailhead at Elbow Fork or Big Water.

DOGS: Must be leashed on even-numbered days; can be unleashed on odd-numbered days

GPS TRAILHEAD COORDINATES

N40° 41.493´ W111° 40.222´

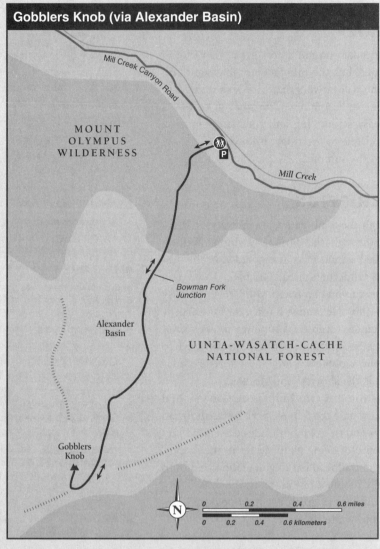

Gobblers Knob (via Alexander Basin)

Mill Creek Canyon Road

MOUNT
OLYMPUS
WILDERNESS

Mill Creek

Bowman Fork
Junction

Alexander
Basin

UINTA-WASATCH-CACHE
NATIONAL FOREST

Gobblers
Knob

0   0.2   0.4   0.6 miles

0   0.2   0.4   0.6 kilometers

N

Views into Big Cottonwood Canyon

Nobody lost any time cutting switchbacks when making this trail. It shoots directly up the center of the basin and follows a steep track throughout. If you keep a steady pace, you should be at the Bowman Fork junction within 30–40 minutes. At this point you've already covered 0.9 mile and gained more than 1,100 feet in elevation. The Bowman Fork Trail drops down and to your right, but you should continue straight ahead. In another 0.2 mile, the woods thin and the trail opens to views leading up the basin.

In late spring and early summer, wildflowers line the trail every step of the way—even on the rocky upper slopes—but they're most abundant in the woods and in the open areas of the upper basin. Larkspur, cow parsnip, phlox, and blue-bells flourish, and you'll spot the elegant and rare white columbine both in the woods and in the open fields.

Alexander Basin is a stairway of tiered basins leading to an upper bowl. Until you reach the middle of the upper bowl, which is covered with patches of snow into midsummer, the trail proves easy to follow. As you stand in the upper bowl, looking up to the rim, you'll see Gobblers Knob on the right side of the rim. From this point you may have to improvise a bit, but you can usually spot a faint route leading up through the subalpine fir in the bowl's center, or alternatively, another faint cairned route leading up the rocky slope to the right of the trees. If it's at all muddy, choose the rocky slope. Either way, the route will be steep leading to the same destination—the bowl's rim.

Once there, you'll overlook the green expanse of Big Cottonwood Canyon, including many of the prominent peaks along the ridge. From this rim vantage

White columbine

point, look down and make a mental note of your route up the bowl so you'll have a reliable return route.

Now it's just a short climb to the Gobblers Knob summit, on a faint but discernible trail leading up to the west and north along craggy slopes. From the rim it's just 10 minutes of sustained climbing on the dry south-facing slope to the summit. While you can see large slices of the Salt Lake Valley from the top of Gobblers Knob, many of the peaks at the Wasatch's western front block the view. Instead, focus on the most impressive views: the peaks along the southern ridge of Big Cottonwood Canyon and to the east.

Cliff swallows and mountain bluebirds dart in and out of the fir and limber pine at the summit. As you descend to the ridge, look to the west and you'll see a well-worn path leading along the ridge toward Mount Raymond. From the ridge, this trail leads back down to the Terrace Campground and the Bowman Fork trailhead in Mill Creek Canyon. A wonderful trail, this path is well worth taking if you have a shuttle vehicle waiting or don't mind hiking an additional 3.5 miles up Mill Creek Canyon to your car.

NEARBY ACTIVITIES

Big Water is Mill Creek Canyon's Grand Central Station and provides easy access to many of the upper canyon's most popular hikes. The two large Big Water parking areas at the top of the canyon provide easy access to the Great Western Trail, Little Water Trail, and Lower Big Water Trail. These lots, which often fill on weekends, are also popular with cyclists who find Big Water the perfect jumping-off point for the expansive network of trails.

MILL CREEK TO PARK CITY OVERLOOK (including Murdock Peak)

IN BRIEF

A gently ascending trail leads along the upper section of Mill Creek to a ridgeline at the top of the canyon. Enjoy the overview at the saddle or continue up to Murdock Peak for the view from the summit.

DESCRIPTION

Well known and well used by locals, Mill Creek Canyon offers wonderful year-round recreational opportunities for hikers, dog owners, road and mountain bikers, cross-country skiers, and snowshoers. Even the farthest reaches of the canyon can get busy on summer weekends. The Upper Big Water trailhead is such a place, with a large parking area that often fills to capacity. But once you get on this trail, the wooded creeksides and the rolling hillsides make the upper canyon a place of serenity.

Big Water Gulch offers plenty of trail options and potential destinations. This less-traveled but particularly enjoyable trail heads directly east from the upper parking area and follows Mill Creek to its headwaters, connects to the Great Western Trail, and ascends the ridge overlooking Park City. If a summit destination is what you have in mind, you can climb to a higher overlook or even continue to the summit of Murdock Peak.

Directions ⟶

From I-215 on Salt Lake City's east side, take the 3300 South/3900 South turnoff (Exit 4). Turn left onto Wasatch Boulevard and go north 1 block to 3800 South. Turn right on 3800 South and continue toward the mouth of Mill Creek Canyon. Pass the toll booth at 0.7 mile and continue another 8.5 miles to the end of Mill Creek Canyon Road. Park in the Upper Big Water trailhead parking area.

KEY AT-A-GLANCE INFORMATION

LENGTH: 5.2 miles round-trip to ridgeline saddle, 6.6 miles round-trip to summit of Murdock Peak

ELEVATION GAIN: 1,177' to ridgeline saddle, 1,979' to Murdock Peak

ELEVATION AT TRAILHEAD: 7,623'

CONFIGURATION: Out-and-back

DIFFICULTY: Moderate

SCENERY: Wooded trail with meadows and rounded peaks; ridgeline and summit views to the east

EXPOSURE: Mostly shaded

TRAFFIC: Moderate

TRAIL SURFACE: Dirt

HIKING TIME: 2–4 hours

WATER REQUIREMENTS: 1–2 liters; water in creek can be purified.

SEASON: Summer–early fall. Gate to upper Mill Creek Canyon is closed November 1–July 1.

ACCESS: Mill Creek Canyon is a fee-access area within Uinta-Wasatch-Cache National Forest (see page 4).

MAPS: USGS Mount Aire, Park City West; Trails Illustrated, Wasatch Front (709)

FACILITIES: Restrooms and drinking water at trailhead

DOGS: Must be leashed on even-numbered days; can be unleashed on odd-numbered days

GPS TRAILHEAD COORDINATES

N40° 41.083′ W111° 38.815′

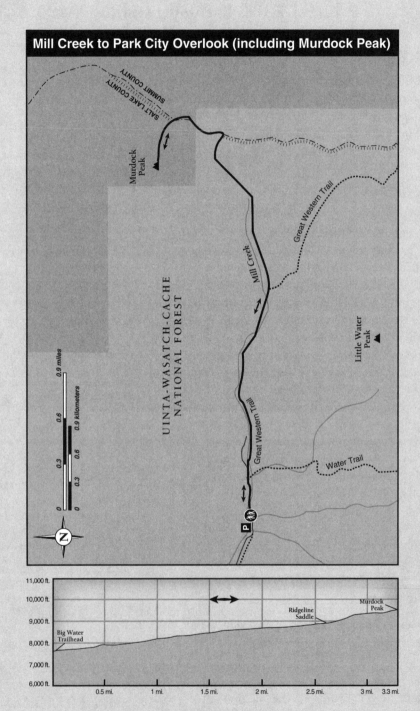

Mill Creek to Park City Overlook (including Murdock Peak)

Bull moose on the Great Western Trail

Departing on the main trail to the east, known both as Mill Creek Trail and Red Pine Road, follow the route along the creek to a fork. Even though the sign points to a trail on the right, take the less-crowded hiking trail on the left. This will hug the creek bank in a deeply wooded section of the canyon and take you away from the mountain bikers who use the wider trail, on the right. This secluded section of trail is soft dirt carpeted with spruce needles, providing a great walking surface for dogs.

At 0.8 mile, the trail crosses the creek over stepping-stones, then within 0.1 mile crosses again to the south side. At 1.2 miles, the trail crests and drops slightly into a meadow ringed with Douglas-fir and shimmering aspens.

Within a few minutes you'll connect with the Great Western Trail. Although the sign at the junction may seem confusing, go left in the direction of Desolation Lake. This will lead you eastward to the ridge overlooking Park City, at which point the trail eventually turns south toward Desolation Lake.

This section of the Great Western Trail is wide and well traveled, with room for both mountain bikers and hikers. Still, be alert, as mountain bikes can often descend the trail at high speeds and come up on you without warning. Morning hikers may well share the trail with moose and deer, who find a hospitable habitat in these moist meadows.

At 2.2 miles, the landscape opens up to high meadows, grassy aspen-covered slopes, and rounded hilltops—very different from the Wasatch canyons to the south.

Ridgeline views from Park City overlook

As the trail continues its gentle ascent, you arrive almost without warning at the 8,800-foot ridgeline saddle. The Great Western Trail turns south toward Big Cottonwood Canyon and Desolation Lake. Continuing eastward for just another 100 feet gives you a nice view of Park City below. But a quick glance to your left reveals the ridgeline leading up to the higher overlook on the way to Murdock Peak.

No real trail takes you to the higher unnamed overlook, or even to Murdock Peak, but the route is clear and the bushwhacking along game trails through low-lying sage and juniper is easy. At a steady pace you'll arrive at the first overlook about 10 minutes after leaving the saddle. From the 9,300-foot overlook, you're above the Park City ski lifts and have a sweeping view of the valley below.

Another 10–15 minutes and 300 feet of elevation gain will put you on the summit of Murdock Peak, along the ridge to the west. While the overlook and the summit are both rewarding destinations, the most beautiful parts of the hike can be found in the meadows, gentle slopes, and wooded creeksides of the upper canyon.

NEARBY ACTIVITIES

Park City Mountain Resort is a premier summer and winter destination just 30 minutes east of Salt Lake City. Summer attractions include an alpine slide, the elevated alpine coaster, an exhilarating zipline, and lift-assisted hiking and mountain biking. For information, visit **parkcitymountain.com**.

NEFFS CANYON 23

IN BRIEF

This spur canyon just south of Mill Creek Canyon has led its life in the shadows of Mount Olympus, so its beauty and history are often overlooked. The steep trail ascends along one of the many canyon streams to a high aspen-ringed meadow surrounded by towering peaks.

DESCRIPTION

The canyons that slice through the Wasatch Mountains not only provided water to the Salt Lake Valley but also powered many of its early industries. One 1847 Mormon pioneer, John Neff, brought his milling machinery with him to the Salt Lake Valley. He built the first mill in the valley at the mouth of Mill Creek, and by 1848 he was producing flour. In his lifetime he built 30 mills, including one near the canyon that bears his name.

Today the Olympus Cove neighborhood has grown up around the access point to Neffs Canyon, and only locals regularly use the trailhead. In all likelihood, fewer people know about Neffs Canyon today than 150 years ago, when it was a hotbed of mining, timber, and

---

Directions →

From I-215 on Salt Lake City's east side, take the 3300 South/3900 South turnoff (Exit 4). Turn left onto Wasatch Boulevard and go north 1 block to 3800 South. Turn right onto Wasatch Boulevard and continue south to Oakview Drive (4275 South), marked by an overhead pedestrian bridge. Turn left on Oakview Drive and continue 1.2 miles east to Zarahemla Drive. Turn left on Zarahemla Drive, continue north 0.3 mile to Park Terrace Drive, and turn right. Continue 0.1 mile and turn right onto White Way. Continue 0.2 mile to the trailhead parking area, at the end of White Way.

KEY AT-A-GLANCE INFORMATION

LENGTH: 5.5 miles round-trip

ELEVATION GAIN: 2,445'

ELEVATION AT TRAILHEAD: 5,624'

CONFIGURATION: Out-and-back

DIFFICULTY: Hard

SCENERY: Wooded canyon, meadow with surrounding peaks

EXPOSURE: Mostly shaded

TRAFFIC: Light

TRAIL SURFACE: Dirt, rock

HIKING TIME: 4–5 hours

WATER REQUIREMENTS: 1–2 liters; water from stream can be purified.

SEASON: Year-round

ACCESS: No fees or permits. Gate near trailhead parking area closed 10 p.m.–6 a.m. Much of the hike lies within the Mount Olympus Wilderness Area.

MAPS: USGS Sugar House and Mount Aire, Trails Illustrated Wasatch Front (709)

FACILITIES: No restrooms at trailhead or on trail

DOGS: Permitted. (Note that Neffs Canyon is not a city watershed.)

SPECIAL COMMENTS: Neffs Canyon is a great snowshoe destination, but stay in the lower canyon where the routes aren't so steep and rocky.

GPS TRAILHEAD COORDINATES

N40° 40.620´ W111° 46.578´

Wild roses at the mouth of Neffs Canyon

grazing activity. The mills, mining, and timber operations have been gone for nearly 100 years, but you can still see one of the old millstones at the Utah State Capitol, along with other pioneer relics.

Standing at the trailhead looking up the canyon, you can tell that it's going to be a beautiful setting. What you can't discern is the number of natural springs that dot the canyon, the various routes taken by the streams, and the water flow's steep gradient.

From the large parking area, take the well-marked trail to the east, which rises quickly to a graded service road in just 100 feet. This road continues a gentle incline along the north side of the canyon, passing a water tank on the left at 0.3 mile. At 0.5 mile, the graded road ends as it comes to a wide stream crossing, where you can easily step across on rocks without ever getting wet. After the crossing, the trail continues up the canyon on an old roadbed used by wagons more than 100 years ago. At 1.1 miles, the old roadbed ends and the trail continues as a steep singletrack through Gambel oak and bigtooth maple.

Because of the canyon's long history, dozens of trails follow its springs and streams. Worth exploring, these trails lead through some beautiful conifer wooded areas. If you find yourself on the south side of the canyon, on a faint trail, and up against a rock slab, you're on your own. You'll enjoy nice overlooks and some great rock climbing, but it's not the main trail to the meadow. Although the road may not be the most romantic route, it is reliable and easy to follow. The Neff Canyon Trail doesn't believe in switchbacks, and even if it did, there's not much room for them in this narrow canyon.

At 1.5 miles, the trail enters the Mount Olympus Wilderness Area. The trail, by now a well-worn dirt track, steepens considerably. After climbing steadily through spruce and fir, the trail crosses the stream over a log bridge at 1.8 miles. As the trail gains elevation, you enter large stands of quaking aspens blended with conifers and maples.

Eventually, the steep ascent lets up just a bit as the trail reaches the crest and enters the meadow at 2.5 miles. Another 0.2 mile and you're at the upper, eastern end of the meadow. Bounded by a dense aspen forest on the south, you have perfect views of Mount Raymond and Hobbs Peak above the aspens.

Another little-known feature on one of the slabs to the south of the meadow is Neffs Canyon Cave, a National Natural Landmark. At 1,165 feet, it's one of the deepest caves in the United States. An extremely dangerous cave with most passages dipping steeply at a 45- to 60-degree slope, it has been locked by the U.S. Forest Service. The USFS grants admission only to experienced cavers.

The meadow is a great place for a snack or to sit quietly and watch for wildlife—especially deer, moose, and elk—as it comes to the stream at the south side of the meadow. The return to the trailhead takes about 1.5 hours. From the meadow you can also follow the trail as it curves to the north. Within a mile it intersects the Thayne Canyon Trail, which descends into Mill Creek.

NEARBY ACTIVITIES

On the northeast side of the trailhead parking area is a well and pumping station for **Mount Olympus Spring Water.** The water, which was originally bottled in 1899, is low in dissolved solids and high in oxygen, with a slightly sweet taste. Stainless-steel tankers transport the water from Neffs Canyon to a bottling plant in Salt Lake City. From there, it's distributed to offices, homes, and retail outlets throughout the Mountain West.

MOUNT OLYMPUS 24

IN BRIEF

Mount Olympus is the best-known and most recognizable peak on Salt Lake City's eastern skyline. Geologically, it's a mammoth anticline of purple quartzite slabs jutting out nearly a mile above the valley floor. Physically, it's a steep, demanding trail capped by a Class 3 scramble to the rocky summit, where exceptional views await.

DESCRIPTION

Many locals assign mythic proportions to a Mount Olympus climb. Its foreboding, craggy summit appears to be unclimbable from the valley floor. Typically, it's not the final rock scramble but the steep trail to the saddle that eliminates unconditioned and unprepared hikers. How you handle the trail's first 100 yards best predicts whether you'll make it to the summit. That initial stretch accurately represents the entire trail in terms of steepness. If you need to stop for a rest after 100 yards, multiply that by 60 and you'll have some sense of what the hike entails. As the trail ascends the canyon and leads toward the summit, it becomes more wild and beautiful, but its steep angle doesn't ease up one bit. The trail's lower portions consist of Bonneville Shoreline alluvium studded with quartzite talus and boulders from above.

Directions ⟶

From I-215 on Salt Lake City's east side, go south to 4500 South (Exit 5). Turn left on 4500 South (UT 266), cross over the freeway, and turn right onto Wasatch Boulevard. Drive south 1.6 miles, and turn left onto an unmarked paved road leading up the hillside to a small parking area.

i KEY AT-A-GLANCE INFORMATION

LENGTH: 7 miles round-trip

ELEVATION GAIN: 4,060'

ELEVATION AT TRAILHEAD: 4,966'

CONFIGURATION: Out-and-back

DIFFICULTY: Hard

SCENERY: Exceptional views of the valley with Big Cottonwood Canyon peaks to the south and east

EXPOSURE: Largely exposed to sun for first mile; mostly shaded in canyon for next 2 miles, then mostly exposed on the scramble to the summit

TRAFFIC: Busy

TRAIL SURFACE: Dirt, rock

HIKING TIME: 5–7 hours

WATER REQUIREMENTS: 1–2 liters

SEASON: Late spring, summer, early fall

ACCESS: No fees or permits. Hike lies within the Mount Olympus Wilderness Area.

MAPS: USGS Sugar House, Trails Illustrated Wasatch Front (709)

FACILITIES: No water or toilets at trailhead; water at creek can be purified.

DOGS: Permitted. (Note that Tolcats Canyon is not a city watershed.)

GPS TRAILHEAD COORDINATES

N40° 39.115′ W111° 48.373′

Mount Olympus

Mount Olympus

saddle

0.6 miles
0.6 kilometers
0.4
0.4
0.2
0.2
0

MOUNT OLYMPUS WILDERNESS

Wasatch Boulevard

215

215

9,000 ft.
8,000 ft.
7,000 ft.
6,000 ft.
5,000 ft.
4,000 ft.

Mount Olympus
Saddle

Tolcats Canyon

0.5 mi.   1 mi.   1.5 mi.   2 mi.   2.5 mi.   3 mi.   3.5 mi.

Mount Olympus viewed from the north

Because the Mount Olympus Trail begins just a stone's throw from I-215, you may find it disturbing to hear the roar of freeway traffic in a federally protected wilderness area. But that disturbance lasts for only the first mile or so.

At 0.5 mile the trail curves to the left around a quartzite outcrop, then proceeds up Tolcats Canyon to the east. At 0.7 mile the path enters the Mount Olympus Wilderness Area, marked by a sign. Eventually, at a point fairly deep in the canyon and 1.7 miles from the trailhead, you'll cross a small creek. The crossing's elevation is 6,256 feet, a 1,290-foot gain from the trailhead. The shade and boulders surrounding the creek make it a popular rest stop.

Beyond the creek crossing, the trail continues its steep ascent to the head of the canyon, aided by several series of switchbacks. Deep in the canyon, at 2.4 miles from the trailhead, conifers begin to appear, and at higher elevations stands of aspen line the trail. This section of trail is particularly beautiful, rocky, and steep.

Soon you approach the saddle, at an elevation of 8,400 feet. The trail levels and turns north through a peaceful grove of Douglas-fir. Take a minute and walk 20 feet or so over to the eastern side of the saddle. The view to the east, a maze of rocky crags, looks absolutely inaccessible and deserving of the wilderness designation.

Because of the trail's popularity and its proximity to the city, wildlife sightings are rare—but rattlesnakes appear fairly often, both on the trail and on the lower sections of the summit scramble. As you're climbing through this area, use caution when placing your hand on rocky ledges so as not to surprise a rattler.

From the saddle, follow the trail north toward the summit. Within 100 yards of traversing the saddle, the grove of Douglas-fir gives way to rocky slopes, and soon you'll be climbing hand over hand. The trail becomes faint, but with some careful scouting, it's generally discernible. No exceptionally difficult or technical movements are required, so if you come to an insurmountable point, retrace your steps and relocate the trail. The route from the saddle to the summit entails 15–20 minutes of sustained scrambling. This section is prone to rockfall, so be careful not to dislodge rocks onto climbers below.

The summit of Mount Olympus consists of an enormous rockpile of angular quartzite boulders. As you'd expect, spectacular views of the Salt Lake Valley await. On a clear day, they extend far up the Great Salt Lake to the northwest and to Deseret Peak in the distant west. The views of the Twin Peaks Wilderness to the south are equally striking.

Mount Olympus's summit is the last place you want to be if the weather forecast calls for lightning. Do not attempt the summit if there is any chance of lightning or rain. Remember that descending from the rocky summit is generally more dangerous and more time-consuming than the climb up. Take your time and save your strength for the jarring downhill return.

Note: No motorized vehicles or bicycles are permitted within the Mount Olympus Wilderness Area. The trailhead parking area accommodates just 18 cars; on busy summer weekends, overflow parking is available on Wasatch Boulevard.

NEARBY ACTIVITIES

Just 5 miles from the Mount Olympus trailhead, **Wheeler Historic Farm** in Salt Lake City (6351 S. 900 East) offers tours, tractor rides, wagon rides, and demonstrations of agriculture and Salt Lake County's rural lifestyle from 1890 to 1920. Open year-round; for more information, call 801-264-2241 or visit **wheelerfarm.com.**

DOG LAKE 25

IN BRIEF

A small, peaceful lake ringed by quaking aspens lies at the junction of several trails leading to other peaks and canyons. A well-used mountain-biking trail, the Dog Lake Trail is wide and easy to follow.

DESCRIPTION

Dog Lake, which lies within Big Cottonwood Canyon, is both remote and accessible, out-of-the-way yet easy to find. It can easily be accessed from Mill D North Fork (as described here) or Butler Fork in the Mount Olympus Wilderness Area. It is also frequently accessed from Mill Creek Canyon. If you're armed with a good trail map of the area, it's easy to plan a canyon-to-canyon hike with Dog Lake as the centerpiece.

A hike to Dog Lake from Big Cottonwood's Mill D North Fork is one of the few trails in the Wasatch without a single switchback. In a little more than 2 miles, the trail ascends steadily but never too steeply. Because of its gradual incline, the trail is popular with mountain bikers. Hikers also love the wide, easily followed trail, which readily accommodates those who want to chat and walk side-by-side. Because the route cuts through aspen

KEY AT-A-GLANCE INFORMATION

LENGTH: 4.6 miles round-trip

ELEVATION GAIN: 1,452'

ELEVATION AT TRAILHEAD: 7,295'

CONFIGURATION: Out-and-back or one-way connecting to other area trails

DIFFICULTY: Easy

SCENERY: Wooded canyon and lake

EXPOSURE: Mostly shaded

TRAFFIC: Moderate

TRAIL SURFACE: Dirt

HIKING TIME: 2–3 hours

WATER REQUIREMENTS: 1 liter; water from stream and lake can be purified.

SEASON: Late spring, summer, early fall

ACCESS: No fees or permits

MAPS: USGS Mount Aire, Trails Illustrated Wasatch Front (709)

FACILITIES: Restrooms across the street from trailhead

DOGS: Prohibited in Big Cottonwood Canyon, a protected watershed

SPECIAL COMMENTS: You'll be sharing the trail with cyclists, as this is a popular mountain-biking trail.

Directions

From Salt Lake City's east side, take I-215 south to 6200 South (Exit 6). At the off-ramp, turn left and proceed south 1.7 miles, as 6200 South changes to Wasatch Boulevard (UT 190). Turn left at the signal, staying on UT 190, and continue 9.1 miles up Big Cottonwood Canyon to the Mill D North Fork trailhead and parking area, on the left side of the road.

GPS TRAILHEAD COORDINATES

N40° 38.978´ W111° 38.893´

Dog Lake

Dog Lake

and meadows, visibility is good, allowing hikers and bikers to see one another on its long, straight stretches.

From the Mill D North Fork trailhead, the trail quickly ascends to the north, then immediately turns right to rise parallel to the canyon road on your right. The trail parallels the road for 0.4 mile before curving to the left and entering Mill D North Fork. At this point the trail is already far above the canyon floor, and it maintains a gentle ascent for another 0.8 mile until it joins with Mill D Creek.

Mill D has more-moderate and less-rugged slopes than other Big Cottonwood side canyons. While it's not as dramatic or rocky, it is beautiful, especially in fall as the aspens turn bright yellow. In the summer, daisies and alpine asters line the path.

At 1.7 miles from the trailhead, you arrive at a signed junction and the Desolation Trail. The path to the right leads to Desolation Lake. Take the route to the left, which takes you directly to Dog Lake, just 0.6 mile farther. This trail leads through more aspens sprinkled with Douglas-fir. As you near the lake, the gradient increases a bit, but never long enough to become tiring. With a steady pace you should arrive at Dog Lake, which lies at an elevation of 8,544 feet, about an hour after you leave the trailhead.

A still, shallow, circular basin ringed by aspen and conifers, Dog Lake may be too small to be called a lake and too large to be called a pond. Because it's shielded from wind, the lake typically has a glassy surface that reflects the surrounding trees like a flawless mirror. Bring your camera, walk around the lake, and enjoy the peaceful setting.

At the north end of the lake is a marked junction on the Desolation Trail. Continuing to the west for 2.8 miles will lead down Butler Fork and back to Big Cottonwood Canyon. From the Butler Fork trailhead, it's just 0.8 mile up the canyon road back to the Mill D North Fork trailhead. If you're adventurous and energetic, take the Big Water Trail over the ridge into Mill Creek Canyon. It's a scenic route, but unless you have a shuttle vehicle awaiting you, it could be a long walk back to your car.

NEARBY ACTIVITIES

Storm Mountain is the imposing barrier that sits 2.5 miles up Big Cottonwood Canyon and made access to the canyon so difficult for early pioneers. **Stairs Gulch** is a short 0.5-mile hike up a rocky couloir at the base of the mountain. To access the trail, park near the geology sign on the right side of the road 100 yards beyond the Storm Mountain Picnic Area. Follow the trail up and to the west before turning south into Stairs Gulch.

DESOLATION LAKE

IN BRIEF

A gentle canyon trail ascends to a high-alpine lake, then leads to a ridge overlooking Park City and Big Cottonwood Canyon. A steep descent of a little-known canyon returns you to the Big Cottonwood Canyon floor.

DESCRIPTION

The 17-mile Desolation Trail stretches from the mouth of Mill Creek Canyon to the top of Big Cottonwood Canyon—from canyon floor to ridgeline. While few hikers ever follow the complete trail from end to end, sections of this scenic trail are popular as a means of connecting various canyons, lakes, and trailheads.

A hike to Desolation Lake—labeled as Lake Desolation on USGS maps—is an excellent orientation hike to Big Cottonwood Canyon because it leads hikers through two side canyons (Mill D North Fork and Beartrap Fork), ascends a panoramic ridgeline, and affords a stop at Desolation Lake. Dog Lake can also be included in the hike by means of a short side trip.

From the Mill D North Fork trailhead, you'll ascend quickly to the north, then immediately turn right to rise parallel to the canyon road on your right. The trail parallels the road for 0.4 mile before curving left and entering

KEY AT-A-GLANCE INFORMATION

LENGTH: 6.6 miles + 1.6 miles by shuttle or on foot

ELEVATION GAIN: 2,465'

ELEVATION AT TRAILHEAD: 7,295'

CONFIGURATION: One-way or loop

DIFFICULTY: Moderate

SCENERY: Canyons, alpine lake, ridgeline views

EXPOSURE: Mostly shaded

TRAFFIC: Moderate

TRAIL SURFACE: Dirt, rock

HIKING TIME: 3–4 hours

WATER REQUIREMENTS: 1–2 liters; water in lake and streams can be purified.

SEASON: Spring, summer, fall

ACCESS: No fees or permits

MAPS: USGS Mount Aire, Park City West, Trails Illustrated Wasatch Front (709)

FACILITIES: Restrooms across the street from trailhead

DOGS: Prohibited in Big Cottonwood Canyon, a protected watershed.

SPECIAL COMMENTS: You'll be sharing the trail with cyclists, as Mill D North Fork and the Desolation Trail are popular mountain-biking trails. The descent down Beartrap Fork is more secluded.

Directions

From Salt Lake City's east side, take I-215 south to 6200 South (Exit 6). At the off-ramp, turn left and proceed south 1.7 miles, as 6200 South changes to Wasatch Boulevard (UT 190). Turn left at the signal, staying on UT 190, and continue 9.1 miles up Big Cottonwood Canyon to the Mill D North Fork trailhead and parking area, on the left side of the road.

GPS TRAILHEAD COORDINATES

N40° 38.978´ W111° 38.893´

Desolation Lake

Photo: Rob Wirt

Desolation Lake in winter

Mill D North Fork. At this point the trail is already far above the canyon floor, and it maintains a gentle ascent for another 0.8 mile until it joins Mill D Creek.

As you ascend Mill D, you'll notice that the slopes on both sides of the canyon are more moderate and less rugged than slopes in other Big Cottonwood side canyons. While Mill D is not particularly dramatic or rocky, it is beautiful, especially in fall as the aspens turn bright yellow. In the summer, daisies and alpine asters line the path.

At 1.7 miles from the trailhead, you arrive at a signed junction and the Desolation Trail. Before continuing on the path to the right, which leads to Desolation Lake, consider a side trip to Dog Lake, just 0.6 mile farther along the path to your left. The Dog Lake option will add another 30 minutes and 1.2 miles to your trip.

From the junction, continue another 1.9 miles along the north slope of a small canyon as it leads through aspens in its ascent to Desolation Lake. The lake lies at an elevation of 9,232 feet in a broad, shallow bowl ringed by a treeless shoreline—hence the *desolation* moniker. In actuality, the meadow to the north and the trees

Trail through aspens from Mill D to Desolation Lake

on the upper slopes create a peaceful openness that is anything but desolate. It's not uncommon to see deer and elk feeding near Desolation Lake.

A trail ringing the lake makes a pleasant extension if you want to visit the woods at the south side of the lake. From the north side, you can turn around and retrace your ascent route to return to the Mill D North Fork trailhead, or you can continue up to the ridge on the east for an interesting variation leading back to Big Cottonwood Canyon.

From Desolation Lake, take the trail from the northeast shore of the lake as it leads up to the ridgeline along an extended switchback. Within a few minutes, you'll be at the top of the ridge on the Great Western Trail leading toward Guardsman Pass and approaching a jagged section popularly known among mountain bikers as "the spine." Along this ridge you'll have fine views down into Park City to the east. Passing the spine, the trail leads south to the right of a knoll and continues along a level contour. As the Great Western Trail begins to curve to the left, you'll notice a faint, unmarked trail that leads to the southwest, down a grassy slope into a canyon. This is Beartrap Fork, a quiet side canyon on the north side of Big Cottonwood.

Continuing down the trail, you will soon connect with a seasonal creekbed at the bottom of Beartrap Canyon. Follow this creek as it leads toward the floor of Big Cottonwood Canyon. The total distance from the Great Western Trail junction through Beartrap Fork down to Big Cottonwood Canyon is 2.2 miles. Once you arrive at the canyon floor and near the road, you'll pass through a metal gate, but no signs indicate that you've just descended Beartrap Fork. Unless you've left a shuttle vehicle at the Beartrap Fork gate, you'll need to walk 1.6 miles down the canyon road back to the Mill D North Fork trailhead.

NEARBY ACTIVITIES

Solitude Mountain Resort, well known for its winter skiing, also offers a varied summer program. Featured activities include lift-served hiking, mountain biking, mountain scooters, disc golf, and casual dining. For information, call 801-534-1400 or visit **skisolitude.com.**

27 MOUNT RAYMOND
(via Butler Fork)

KEY AT-A-GLANCE INFORMATION

LENGTH: 8 miles round-trip

ELEVATION GAIN: 3,071'

ELEVATION AT TRAILHEAD: 7,170'

CONFIGURATION: Out-and-back as described; many one-way, spur, and loop options

DIFFICULTY: Hard

SCENERY: Wooded drainage, aspen slopes, high ridgeline ascent to a 10,241' peak with great views

EXPOSURE: Mostly shaded for first 2 miles, partially shaded to summit

TRAFFIC: Moderate

TRAIL SURFACE: Dirt, rock

HIKING TIME: 4.5–5.5 hours

WATER REQUIREMENTS: 1–2 liters. For the first mile you'll have access to Butler Fork water, which can be purified.

SEASON: Late spring, summer, midfall

ACCESS: No fees or permits

MAPS: USGS Mount Aire, Trails Illustrated Wasatch Front (709)

FACILITIES: No restrooms or water at trailhead

DOGS: Prohibited in Big Cottonwood Canyon, a protected watershed

GPS TRAILHEAD COORDINATES

N40° 38.967´ W111° 39.717´

IN BRIEF

Admittedly, neighboring Gobblers Knob is 5 feet higher in elevation and has a more interesting name, but Mount Raymond is the more interesting hike. Groves of aspen blanket the lower trail, and a variety of conifers clings to a rocky knife-ridge leading to the summit. You'll have great views in all directions.

DESCRIPTION

A hike to the summit of Mount Raymond supplies a great example of the interconnection of many Wasatch trails. As you browse the summit log, you may find that most of the other hikers arrived by some other route. The path described here departs from the Butler Fork Trailhead in Big Cottonwood Canyon, but you could just as easily use the Mill B North Fork trailhead or one of several Mill Creek Canyon trailheads. The Butler Fork route attains the summit with the least vertical ascent, though, and still offers an appealing approach. Along the route to the summit, you'll come to five trail junctions, and while you'll want to explore them all, you may have to save some for another day.

From the small roadside parking area, follow the trail leading north along the west side of a small stream. The trail immediately

---

Directions ⟶

From Salt Lake City's east side, take I-215 south to 6200 South (Exit 6). At the off-ramp, turn left and proceed south 1.7 miles, as 6200 South changes to Wasatch Boulevard (UT 190). Turn left at the signal, staying on UT 190, and continue 8.2 miles up Big Cottonwood Canyon to the small parking area on the left side of the road.

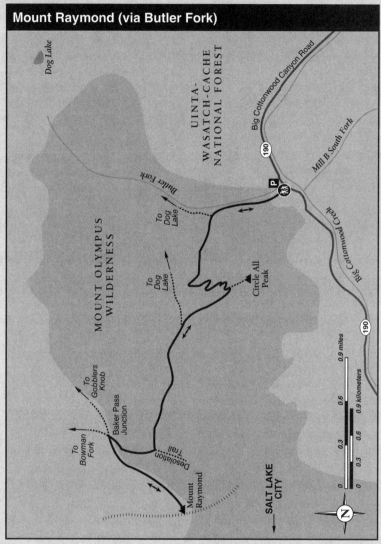

Mount Raymond (via Butler Fork)

Dog Lake

UINTA-WASATCH-CACHE NATIONAL FOREST

Big Cottonwood Canyon Road

190

Mill B South Fork

Butler Fork

P

Big Cottonwood Creek

To Dog Lake

Circle All Peak

To Dog Lake

MOUNT OLYMPUS WILDERNESS

190

0.9 miles

To Gobblers Knob

Baker Pass Junction

To Bowman Fork

Desolation Trail

SALT LAKE CITY

Mount Raymond

0.6   0.9 kilometers

0.3   0.6

0   0.3

0

Z

12,000 ft.
11,000 ft.
10,000 ft.   Mount Raymond
9,000 ft.   Baker Pass
8,000 ft.
Butler Fork
7,000 ft.
            1 mi.   2 mi.   3 mi.   4 mi.

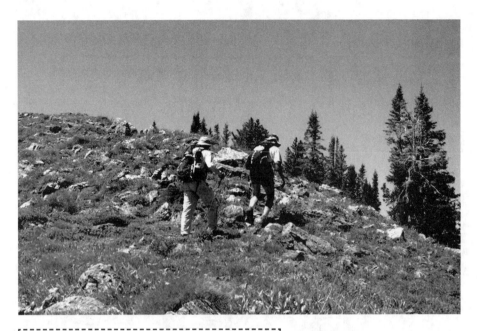

Hikers make their final ascent to Mount Raymond's summit.

crosses to the east side of the stream and enters the Mount Olympus Wilderness Area, marked by a large U.S. Forest Service sign. At 0.5 mile from the trailhead, you'll come to a junction marked by a small USFS sign indicating a trail to Dog Lake on the right and Mill A Basin on the left. Go to the left, up into the aspen-lined drainage.

Within 100 yards, the aspens give way to a clearing about the size of a football field. This area will be your best chance to see moose, especially in the early morning. Never approach a moose—instead, try to work your way around it or wait for it to move. Never come between a moose cow and her calf or between a moose and the water.

From the clearing, the trail continues up the slope through a series of switchbacks. At 1.6 miles from the trailhead, you arrive at a saddle. A faint trail, normally blocked by fallen limbs to steer hikers along the main trail, takes off to the left. It leads to Circle All Peak, an 8,707-foot outcrop overlooking Big Cottonwood Canyon and also Mount Raymond. It's just 0.2 mile to the viewpoint and an elevation gain of 150 feet from the junction. It's certainly worth 10 minutes of your time, and if you're rushed for time it could be a suitable alternate destination for a hike of less than 2 hours.

Back on the main trail, continue along a gently ascending slope to another sign pointing to Dog Lake on the right and Mill A on the left. Follow the trail left as it sweeps along the upper slope of the Mill A Basin. This is a particularly enjoyable section of the hike, with excellent views of Mount Raymond directly to the west. These slopes also provide abundant habitat for many birds, including American redstarts and yellow warblers, which you should be able to hear even if you can't see them.

As you near the top of the Mill A Basin, a faint trail, normally unmarked, takes off along a level contour to the west and leads down to the Mill B North Fork Trailhead. Stay to the right as the trail continues another 0.2 mile up to the saddle of Baker Pass.

From Baker Pass (elevation 9,340), you have your first views into Mill Creek Canyon and west to the Great Salt Lake. Four separate trails meet at this pass. If you turn to the right, a fairly straightforward walk ascends 900 feet in 0.8 mile to the summit of Gobblers Knob. To the left, a more rigorous climb ascends 900 feet in 0.6 mile to the summit of Mount Raymond. Many hikers do both on the same hike, and that's certainly an option you can consider. You can bag two summits in one afternoon.

Departing Baker Pass and walking toward Mount Raymond to the west, you pass an amazing variety of conifers, including Douglas-fir, limber pine, bristlecone pine, and subalpine fir. Some are firmly planted in soil, and others cling tenaciously with exposed roots hugging the rocks. The first 0.3 mile from the pass offers some beautiful steep ascents along a grassy alpine ridge trail. Then the trail ends and you're face-to-face with a fractured ridge of angular limestone and quartzite. It's a good scramble with some exposure, but nothing that would demand protective equipment or technical-climbing experience. There's just enough maneuvering to make it fun.

As you might expect, the summit offers excellent views in all directions. You'll enjoy seeing Mount Olympus from the less familiar back side, and Twin Peaks and Dromedary Peak to the south. At the summit you'll find a USGS marker and a summit log. You'll probably share the views with a handful of other hikers and a few interested chipmunks.

Note: The trail lies within the federally protected Mount Olympus Wilderness Area. Pets, horses, bicycles, motorized vehicles, and open campfires are prohibited.

NEARBY ACTIVITIES

Big Cottonwood Canyon trails are known for their steep ascents to towering peaks and shimmering lakes. An enjoyable introduction to the canyon is the **Mill B South Interpretive Trail**, which follows the rushing Big Cottonwood Creek for a 0.7-mile out-and-back. The trail is paved and wheelchair-accessible, and there are restrooms at the trailhead. Start at the Mill B South Fork Trailhead parking lot, just 4.3 miles up the canyon as you enter the S-curves.

28 DOUGHNUT FALLS

KEY AT-A-GLANCE INFORMATION

LENGTH: 1.4 miles round-trip

ELEVATION GAIN: 337'

ELEVATION AT TRAILHEAD: 7,493'

CONFIGURATION: Out-and-back

DIFFICULTY: Easy

SCENERY: Spruce forest, stream, and waterfall

EXPOSURE: Mostly shaded

TRAFFIC: Busy

TRAIL SURFACE: Dirt, rock

HIKING TIME: 1–2 hours

WATER REQUIREMENTS: 1 liter

SEASON: Late spring, summer, early fall

ACCESS: No fees or permits. Gate to trailhead parking closed in winter and early spring.

MAPS: USGS Mount Aire

FACILITIES: Vault toilet at trailhead; no drinking water, but water from stream can be purified.

DOGS: Big Cottonwood Canyon, a protected watershed, prohibits pets and horses.

SPECIAL COMMENTS: The road to the trailhead passes through private property with NO TRESPASSING signs posted. However, public access to the falls has been maintained.

GPS TRAILHEAD COORDINATES

N40° 38.375´ W111° 39.087´

IN BRIEF

Doughnut Falls is unique—a waterfall that plunges through a hole in the rock and into a grotto before cascading down the rocky drainage below. It's a short hike, popular with families and youth groups. If you want to climb to the top of the falls, you'll face a challenging but rewarding scramble.

DESCRIPTION

Doughnut Falls is irresistible. In less than a mile of easy walking, you come to a rocky chasm with a waterfall that drops through a hole in the rock. The sight is so intriguing that you are compelled to climb as close as possible to see where all that water goes.

As you drive up Big Cottonwood Canyon, you'll notice signs referring to Mill B, Mill C, and so on. This naming system dates back to the 1850s, when the side canyons in Big Cottonwood Canyon were named alphabetically, A–F, with a lumber mill placed at the mouth of each canyon. Doughnut Falls is on the Mill D South Fork. As you drive up the canyon to the trailhead, the canyon widens into a large, open meadow called Reynolds Flat, site of the Jordan Pines picnic area.

After a visitor fell through Doughnut Falls to his death in 1990, signs directing

Directions

From Salt Lake City's east side, take I-215 south to 6200 South (Exit 6). At the off-ramp, turn left and proceed south 1.7 miles, as 6200 South changes to Wasatch Boulevard (UT 190). Turn left at the signal, staying on UT 190, and continue 9 miles up Big Cottonwood Canyon. Turn right at the Jordan Pines picnic area and continue 0.8 mile to the trailhead parking area, on the left.

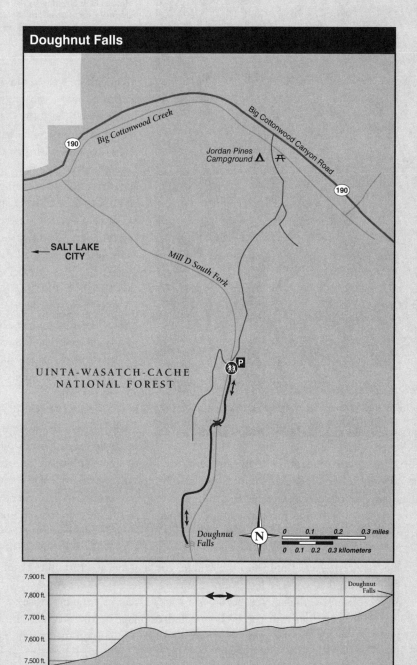

Doughnut Falls

Big Cottonwood Creek

190

Big Cottonwood Canyon Road

190

Jordan Pines
Campground △ ⅂⅄

← SALT LAKE
   CITY

Mill D South Fork

UINTA-WASATCH-CACHE
NATIONAL FOREST

Doughnut
Falls

N

0   0.1   0.2   0.3 miles

0   0.1   0.2   0.3 kilometers

7,900 ft.
7,800 ft.   Doughnut
                                                                        Falls
7,700 ft.
7,600 ft.
7,500 ft.
7,400 ft.
        0.1 mi.   0.2 mi.   0.3 mi.   0.4 mi.   0.5 mi.   0.6 mi.   0.7 mi.

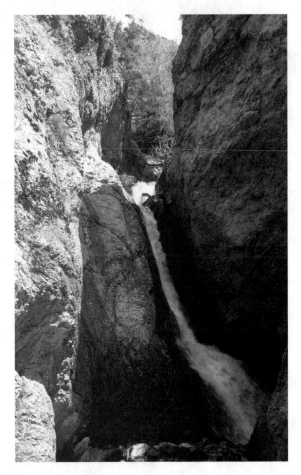

Hidden Falls (see Nearby Activities, opposite, for more information)

people there were removed, giving some visitors the impression that the falls were off-limits. Likewise, some disputes with private-land holders in the area have resulted in a number of PRIVATE PROPERTY and NO TRESPASSING signs being put up, leading some to believe that the falls are closed to the public. In 2007, Salt Lake City purchased Doughnut Falls and about 144 surrounding acres as a watershed. The U.S. Forest Service's management of the area preserves public access to the falls.

From the trailhead parking area, the wide trail leads up the canyon through a forest of white, blue, and yellow spruce, dotted with limber pine and an occasional Douglas-fir. Stands of quaking aspen also brighten the trail, especially in the fall as they turn lemon yellow. At 0.2 mile the wide trail constricts and veers off to the right. At 0.4 mile the trail enters an open area shaded by large conifers. From here, cross the bridge over Mill D South Fork to your right, then immediately turn left onto the old mining road and continue up the canyon with the stream at your left. At 0.1 mile past the bridge, you'll arrive at a fork in the mining road, where you'll stay to the left, following the stream up the canyon.

Almost instantly, the canyon becomes a rocky chasm. By staying close to the stream, you'll be drawn into the boulder-filled drainage below the falls. In the spring, the snow-fed stream spans the chasm, and continuing up toward the falls will require some boulder-hopping and scrambling up steep rock ledges. Getting wet is almost inevitable. In the summer, as the stream flow is reduced, some scrambling will be required, but it's easier to avoid getting wet. Even though Doughnut Falls is a popular family hike, climbing up to the falls may be too hazardous for children younger than age 6.

As you weave through the large boulders below the falls and scale the rocky ledges leading up to them, be sure to stay on the west side of the stream, to the right of the falls. This will give you the safest access and put you face-to-face with the falls' intriguing layout.

Doughnut Falls plunges through a hole about 6 feet in diameter and drops into a grotto about 20 feet long and 10 feet wide. You'll want to get close—and most visitors get within a few feet of the grotto—but be careful. It's easy to spend an hour or more playing around here.

On your way to the falls and back, be on the lookout for moose, who find a luxurious habitat in this drainage. Beaver still appear in the stream, and foxes occasionally dart behind trees. But the most likely sightings will be ground squirrels and chipmunks in a lush home of spruce and aspen.

NEARBY ACTIVITIES

As long as you're visiting Doughnut Falls, don't miss **Hidden Falls** on your way up the canyon. It's only 100 yards from the road and takes just a few minutes to visit. As you come to the S-curve, 4.3 miles up the canyon, enter the Mill B North Fork parking area, 100 yards past the Mill B South Fork parking area. Take the trailhead at the north side of the parking area and cross the road. Rather than following the Mill B North Fork Trail, follow the creek to your left—within a few seconds, Hidden Falls appears as if by magic.

29   LAKE BLANCHE

KEY AT-A-GLANCE INFORMATION

LENGTH: 5.8 miles round-trip

ELEVATION GAIN: 2,670'

ELEVATION AT TRAILHEAD: 6,240'

CONFIGURATION: Out-and-back

DIFFICULTY: Moderate

SCENERY: Canyon with glacial geology, stream, glacial lakes, surrounding peaks

EXPOSURE: Mostly shaded up to lake, then partially shaded

TRAFFIC: Busy

TRAIL SURFACE: Dirt, rock

HIKING TIME: 3.5–5 hours

WATER REQUIREMENTS: 1–2 liters

SEASON: Late spring, summer, early fall; avalanche hazard in winter and early spring

ACCESS: No fees or permits

MAPS: USGS Mount Aire, Dromedary Peak; Trails Illustrated Wasatch Front (709)

FACILITIES: Vault toilet at trailhead; no drinking water, but water from stream and lake can be purified.

DOGS: Prohibited in Big Cottonwood Canyon, a protected watershed

GPS TRAILHEAD COORDINATES

N40° 37.968´ W111° 43.415´

IN BRIEF

Lake Blanche is a classic glacial tarn at the base of a cirque. The hike to Lake Blanche begins at the Big Cottonwood Canyon floor and follows the dramatically glaciated side canyon to an exceptionally scenic and remote alpine setting. It's one of the most popular hikes in the Salt Lake area—and justifiably so.

DESCRIPTION

It's entirely possible to walk out of a meeting in the Fort Union business and financial district and, within 15 minutes, be following a roaring stream up a glacial canyon in a federally designated wilderness area. And that's only the beginning. The highlight, Lake Blanche, awaits under a glacial cirque at the top of the canyon. No wonder this is such a popular hike.

The parking area at the Mill B South Fork trailhead holds 24 cars, but you can also park along the road. The parking lot serves both the Broads Fork trailhead at the west end of the lot and the Mill B South Fork (Lake Blanche) trailhead at the east side of the lot, to the left of the vault toilet. Take this paved trail as it parallels Big Cottonwood Creek to your left. Within about 0.2 mile and just before the paved trail crosses a bridge, the Lake Blanche

---

Directions

From Salt Lake City's east side, take I-215 south to 6200 South (Exit 6). At the off-ramp, turn left and proceed south 1.7 miles, as 6200 South changes to Wasatch Boulevard (UT 190). Turn left at the signal, staying on UT 190, and continue 4.3 miles up Big Cottonwood Canyon. As the road makes a hairpin turn to the left, enter the Mill B South trailhead parking area, on the right.

Lake Blanche

MOUNT OLYMPUS WILDERNESS

190

Big Cottonwood Canyon Road

Big Cottonwood Creek

190

P

UINTA-WASATCH-CACHE NATIONAL FOREST

Broads Fork

Mill B South Fork

TWIN PEAKS WILDERNESS

Lake Florence

Lake Blanche

Lake Lillian

Sundial Peak

N

0   0.4   0.8   1.2 miles

0   0.4   0.8   1.2 kilometers

11,000 ft.

10,000 ft.

9,000 ft.

8,000 ft.

7,000 ft.

6,000 ft.

Lake Blanche

Mill B South Fork

0.5 mi.   1 mi.   1.5 mi.   2 mi.   2.5 mi.   2.9 mi.

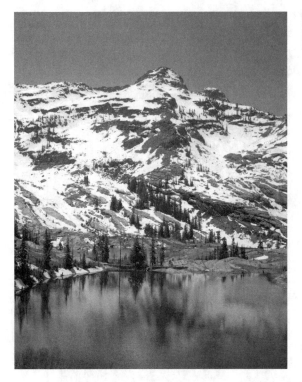

Lake Florence

Trail departs the paved trail, bearing to the right and becoming a rocky path.

After 0.1 mile on the Lake Blanche dirt trail, you'll cross a bridge to the east side of the Mill B South Fork and continue up a switchback to the north. Within another 0.2 mile, you'll enter the Twin Peaks Wilderness Area with the stream at your right as you head up the canyon.

The trail steadily ascends the canyon in a shaded forest. Soon, within the upper area of the canyon, you'll pass through several acres of avalanche damage, where hundreds of trees have been toppled like so many toothpicks. Follow the course of destruction by looking at the release area on the denuded avalanche-prone slope to the west. Observe how the avalanche crossed the stream and took out trees on the opposite slope from where you stand. Above and below the avalanche zone, the trail is largely shaded by a blanket of aspen and dotted with Douglas-fir.

Near the top of Mill B South Fork, you ascend the slope above the aspen to the eastern side of the canyon. Along the high switchbacks, you can catch a narrow glimpse of the Salt Lake Valley through the canyon's mouth. At 2.4 miles from the trailhead, you come to a talus slope composed of quartzite boulders. The trail skirts the large rock pile and continues up to the south. Within 100 yards of the first talus field, the trail crosses another quartzite field.

As you approach the large quartzite formation at the top of the canyon, you'll begin to notice evidence of glacial activity. As glaciers transported rocks and debris over the surface of the formation, they left striations on the quartzite's surface that are still clearly visible.

As you crest the formation, Lake Blanche comes into full view. As you look across the lake, Sundial Peak stands at the center of the cirque. While the quartzite formation forms the northern shore of the lake, the remains of a concrete reinforced rock dam are visible on both sides of the quartzite dome. This dam was built in the 1930s to contain a much larger reservoir. Many of the upper Wasatch lakes were controlled and maintained as reservoirs to ensure a consistent supply

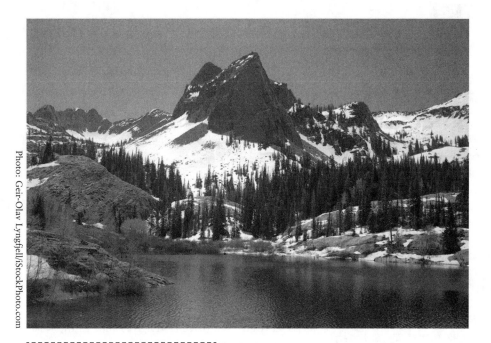

Photo: Geir-Olav Lyngfjell/iStockPhoto.com

Lake Blanche, at the base of Sundial Peak

of water throughout the summer. The Lake Blanche dam broke along the western rim in 1983, leaving the lake at its present size. If you're tempted to take a dip in the icy waters, remember that swimming is not permitted in watershed lakes.

Lake Blanche is a destination resort in the wilderness. Take your time, walk around, study the geology, count the wildflowers, look for waterfalls, and explore the woods at the far end of the lake. Allow at least an hour at and around the lake. As you walk to the western side of Lake Blanche, you'll discover two smaller tarns—Lake Florence and Lake Lillian—in a lower glacial bowl. These more-remote lakes get less traffic, provide a quiet place to rest, and offer better chances for wildlife-viewing.

Note: The Lake Blanche Trail lies within the federally protected Twin Peaks Wilderness Area. Pets, horses, bicycles, motorized vehicles, and open campfires are prohibited.

NEARBY ACTIVITIES

As you drive back down Big Cottonwood Canyon following your hike, you may want to stop at the **Storm Mountain Picnic Area.** Near the picnic sites is the Storm Mountain Amphitheater, which can be reserved for private programs and concerts. The amphitheater holds up to 200 people and offers a dramatic setting for a business or organization event. For reservations, call 801-733-0588.

30 WILLOW HEIGHTS

KEY AT-A-GLANCE INFORMATION

LENGTH: 2 miles round-trip

ELEVATION GAIN: 675'

ELEVATION AT TRAILHEAD: 7,815'

CONFIGURATION: Out-and-back

DIFFICULTY: Easy

SCENERY: Aspen forest, meadows, a quiet lake

EXPOSURE: Mostly shaded

TRAFFIC: Moderate

TRAIL SURFACE: Paved for first 0.2 mile, then dirt to meadow and lake

HIKING TIME: 1–1.5 hours

WATER REQUIREMENTS: 1 liter; water at stream and in lake can be purified.

SEASON: Year-round

ACCESS: No fees or permits

MAPS: USGS Park City West

FACILITIES: No restrooms or water at trailhead

DOGS: Prohibited in Big Cottonwood Canyon, a protected watershed

SPECIAL COMMENTS: Willow Heights is a great snowshoe hike or backcountry ski tour in winter.

GPS TRAILHEAD COORDINATES

N40° 37.928´ W111° 36.518´

IN BRIEF

A short, little-known hike to a high meadow and lake. Situated at the top of Big Cottonwood Canyon, Willow Heights is filled with wildflowers and wildlife, and attracts few people.

DESCRIPTION

You'll find most hikes that lead to lakes in Big Cottonwood Canyon well marked, with ample trailhead parking, and often crowded. Willow Lake has none of these attributes. Because there's no marked trailhead, you'll need to park on the south side of the road (UT 190), cross to a residential drive leading 0.1 mile to the west, then switchback another 0.1 mile to the east. As the pavement ends, the trail begins.

The wide path leads through a hillside of aspen, sprinkled with just a few young fir. Occasionally, the trail steepens, but it's never too strenuous. At 0.8 mile you come to Willow Creek, which can be crossed by the crude bridge of fallen branches or by the stepping-stones several feet upstream.

Within 0.1 mile, the aspen grove opens to a large meadow and views of the upper canyon and ridgeline to the east. As you follow the trail to the upper end of the meadow, you

----

Directions _____→

From Salt Lake City's east side, take I-215 south to 6200 South (Exit 6). At the off-ramp, turn left and proceed south 1.7 miles, as 6200 South changes to Wasatch Boulevard (UT 190). Turn left at the signal, staying on UT 190, and continue 11.1 miles up Big Cottonwood Canyon to Silver Fork Lodge, on the right. Continue another 0.2 mile up the canyon and park on the right side of the road. The trail begins across the street on a narrow, paved road leading to a residential area.

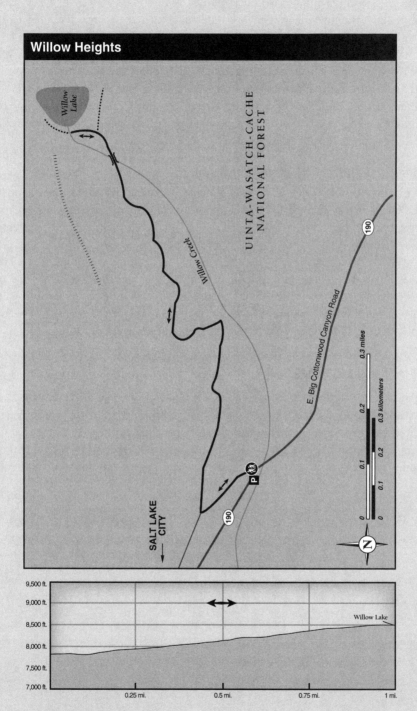

come to a fork. Turning left will lead you to Willow Lake in less than 100 yards. Continuing straight will lead to aptly named Dry Lake, about 0.5 mile to the northeast.

While Willow Lake may be a short hike, don't make it a fast one. Take your time as you approach the lake: explore, walk around the shore, and watch for wildlife. It's the perfect place to spot moose and deer, especially in the early morning and at dusk. A large beaver lodge rises from the middle of the shallow lake, and ducks nest and live near the water in spring and summer. Cliff swallows skim the surface of the lake, and raptors circle high overhead.

Several primitive campsites await on the north side of the lake for those wanting a short hike to a setting of solitude and natural beauty. Willow Lake and the meadow can be buggy in summer, so come prepared with insect repellent.

The meadow and the flatlands around the lake are alive with wildflowers in spring and summer. Phlox is the most abundant, while larkspur and penstemon are also common.

Willow Heights, the open area encompassing both the meadow and the lake, makes a wonderful short morning hike. You can be up to the lake before the sun rises over the ridge, watch the wildlife awaken, and still be back to your nearby lodge or cabin before breakfast. In winter or early spring, a midday snowshoe hike exposes the wildlife as the sun beams through leafless aspen.

NEARBY ACTIVITIES

A great choice for lunch or an extended stay, **Silver Fork Lodge** offers nearby access to skiing, hiking, fishing, and mountain biking. It has a patio and indoor casual dining that you can enjoy without having to get dressed up—even if you've just come off the trail or the ski slopes. The lodge has seven rustic rooms without phones and television, plus an outdoor hot tub. For reservations, call 888-649-9551 or go to **silverforklodge.com.**

JORDAN RIVER PARKWAY

IN BRIEF

The Jordan River Parkway stays close to the river, passing along and through a riparian habitat and floodplain. You can easily reach the trail at dozens of points—parks, street crossings, and residential neighborhoods. When completed, the parkway will extend from the Utah County line to the south to the Davis County line to the north. The section featured here is the longest continuous completed portion and features some of the path's most accessible and enjoyable scenery.

DESCRIPTION

The Jordan River, Utah Lake's outlet, is one of the three major rivers that empty into the Great Salt Lake. Originally named the Utah River, it was renamed by Mormon pioneer Heber C. Kimball, who likened the river to its Holy Land namesake, which also flows from a freshwater lake into an inland salt sea.

The Jordan River Parkway is an ambitious urban trail project that will eventually follow the river throughout Salt Lake County. Presently, the longest completed section of the trail passes through the municipalities of West Jordan, Taylorsville, Murray, and West Valley City, then finally into Salt Lake City. This section can easily be accessed at Gardner Village to the south, at Redwood Trailhead Park to the north, and at dozens of points in between.

The trail snakes its way around the various inlets and marshes that dress the banks of the river, making the trail even more circuitous than the river itself. As the crow flies, this section measures only 7.7 miles in length, but as the trail follows the meandering river, it covers a distance of more than 11 miles. While

KEY AT-A-GLANCE INFORMATION

LENGTH: 11 miles one-way

ELEVATION GAIN: –58' (from beginning to end)

ELEVATION AT TRAILHEAD: 4,290' (Gardner Village), 4,232' (Redwood)

CONFIGURATION: One-way or out-and-back

DIFFICULTY: Easy

SCENERY: Jordan River and surrounding wetlands

EXPOSURE: Partial shade

TRAFFIC: Busy

TRAIL SURFACE: Completely paved and striped

HIKING TIME: Varies greatly based on distance selected

WATER REQUIREMENTS: 0.5 liter–1 liter. You'll find drinking fountains along the trail in most of the parks, as well as restaurants and convenience stores at some nearby street crossings.

SEASON: Year-round

ACCESS: No fees or permits

MAPS: None

FACILITIES: Restrooms, water, phones, and other services at the trailhead and throughout the hike

DOGS: On leash

GPS TRAILHEAD COORDINATES

Gardner Village (south end of trail):
N40° 36.567´ W111° 55.333´
Redwood (north end of trail):
N40° 43.200´ W111° 55.233´

Jordan River Parkway

Directions →

GARDNER VILLAGE TRAILHEAD (south end of trail): Take I-15 south from Salt Lake City to 7200 South (Exit 297). Turn right onto 7200 South (UT 48) toward Midvale. Take the first left onto 700 West. Continue south 0.7 mile on 700 West (Holden Street). Turn right (west) on Center Street and continue 0.5 mile to the Gardner Village entrance, on the right. Access the trail from the Gardner Village parking lot's southeast corner.

REDWOOD TRAILHEAD (north end of trail): Take I-15 south from downtown Salt Lake City to UT 201 (Exit 305A). Continue westbound 1.7 miles on UT 201 and take the Redwood Road exit. At the off-ramp, turn left (south) onto Redwood Road (UT 68). Continue south 0.2 mile and turn left at West 2320 South. Continue east 0.9 mile on West 2320 South. Turn right into the Redwood Trailhead parking area.

  In addition to these starting and ending trailheads, more than a dozen official trailheads supply public parking and easy trail access along the way.

the Jordan does wind and meander, dropping only about 5 feet per mile, it still flows at a surprisingly fast clip.

  Leaving Gardner Village (7800 South), the trail stays on the west bank of the Jordan until 6300 South. As the river flows north, the trail makes several river crossings and also manages to adeptly avoid most major thoroughfares and two freeways with some well-placed underpasses. For the most part, road noise is easy to escape along the trail.

  When early pioneers arrived in the Salt Lake Valley, they noted that the cottonwood- and willow-lined river corridor stood in sharp contrast to the tree-less, sage-covered plains on either side. They soon built settlements along the river and shared the land with wolves and coyotes, while beavers built dams along the river. All are gone today, but foxes, skunks, raccoons, and muskrats still live in the wooded areas near the river.

  More than any other species, you'll see waterfowl. Mallards, grebes, coots, Canada geese, and great blue herons make the parkway marshlands their permanent home. Ring-necked pheasants, chukars, and quail can also be spotted year-round.

  As late as 1910, the riverbanks provided seasonal camping for Ute, Paiute, and Shoshone tribes. Native Americans traded tanned skins and dried meat for supplies. Trailhead markers provide interpretive background on the natural history of the area, as well as insights into pioneer homesteads and early settlements along the river.

  The growth of the Salt Lake Valley, industrialization, dredging, and channeling has not always been kind to the Jordan River. Many of the rich riparian and wetland areas have been lost over the last 100 years. Today, natural-resource damage-settlement funds from the Sharon Steel Superfund Site are being used to restore more than 270 acres of river corridor and floodplain by removing invasive plants, establishing native plants, and contouring some sections of the riverbank.

In addition to waterfowl, chukars can be seen along the parkway.

A number of spur trails and oxbow divisions mark the trail. At some points, the trail divides into a pedestrian portion, while bicycles stay on the paved route. The West Valley City Cross Towne Trail and other spurs connect the main trail to nearby neighborhoods. These poorly marked spurs typically follow a diversion canal or side channel. When in doubt, stay on the trail nearest the river.

North of the Redwood Park Trailhead, the parkway continues unobstructed for another 2 miles, but the surrounding area loses much of its natural beauty and scenic appeal. The setting becomes more industrial with less shade—and for cyclists, more thorns to flatten your tires.

NEARBY ACTIVITIES

Gardner Village, an early-Utah-themed shopping village (1100 W. 7800 South; 801-566-8903; gardnervillage.com), got its start in 1853, when the first flour mill in the South Salt Lake Valley was built on the site. Today, specialty shops, a restaurant, bakery, and day spa cluster in a historic setting, linked by brick paths, gardens, and a covered bridge.

GREAT WESTERN TRAIL
(Guardsman Pass to Clayton Peak)

IN BRIEF

The Great Western Trail is a corridor of trails traversing 4,455 miles through Arizona, Utah, Idaho, Wyoming, and Montana. Within Utah, the Great Western Trail roughly follows the Wasatch ridge running north and south. A short hike from Guardsman Pass to Clayton Peak follows a section of the trail along a scenic ridgeline.

DESCRIPTION

Ridgeline hikes have the benefit of delivering panoramic views and enabling you to put the surrounding peaks and canyons in perspective. This small section of the Great Western Trail demonstrates how interconnected Wasatch canyons are and how easy it is to connect to trails in Park City and Heber Valley to the east. With most of the hike being above 10,000 feet in elevation, there's not much to block the view.

Guardsman Pass offers a high-elevation start for the hike. From the trailhead parking area, take a look around in all directions. Summit County and Park City lie to the north and east, Wasatch County and Heber Valley lie to the south and east, and Big Cottonwood

KEY AT-A-GLANCE INFORMATION

LENGTH: 2.2 miles round-trip

ELEVATION GAIN: 1,015'

ELEVATION AT TRAILHEAD: 9,706'

CONFIGURATION: Out-and-back

DIFFICULTY: Moderate

SCENERY: Mountain scenery, panoramic views

EXPOSURE: Partially shaded

TRAFFIC: Light

TRAIL SURFACE: Dirt, rock

HIKING TIME: 2–2.5 hours

WATER REQUIREMENTS: 1 liter; no water on trail

SEASON: Late spring–early fall

ACCESS: No fees or permits

MAPS: USGS Brighton

FACILITIES: No restrooms or water at trailhead

DOGS: Permitted on trail from pass eastward; prohibited in Big Cottonwood Canyon, a protected watershed, to the west

SPECIAL COMMENTS: This is a great hike for dogs, especially when it includes a loop down into the lakes in the basin to the east..

Directions ⟶

From Salt Lake City's east side, take I-215 south to 6200 South (Exit 6). At the off-ramp, turn left and proceed south 1.7 miles, as 6200 South changes to Wasatch Boulevard (UT 190). Turn left at the signal, staying on UT 190, and continue 13.8 miles up Big Cottonwood Canyon to the Guardsman Pass Road turnoff, on the left. Turn left and continue 3.1 miles up Guardsman Pass Road to the Guardsman Pass parking area, on the right.

GPS TRAILHEAD COORDINATES

N40° 36.402´ W111° 33.297´

A mountainous panorama from Clayton Peak

Canyon lies directly below to the west. The trail leading to Clayton Peak stretches in front of you to the south.

Like most Wasatch trails, this one rises quickly from the trailhead. After less than 30 minutes of hiking at a steady pace, you've already covered 0.6 mile and gained more than 700 feet of elevation. You'll find yourself on top of an unnamed knoll along the ridgeline at an elevation of 10,420 feet. The views are great, but Clayton Peak still looms in the distance to the south. Descend the slope on a faint trail and continue along the ridge, dropping more than 300 feet of hard-earned elevation gain.

Along the way, you can't help but notice the many lakes in the basin to the east. Little-known by most Wasatch hikers, they include Bloods Lake, Lake Brimhall, Silver Lake, Silver Lake Islet, and Lackawaxen Lake. You can reach them by trails leading down from the ridgeline, in particular as part of a loop hike returning to Guardsman Pass.

As you work your way up the ridge, a quick glance to the right will surprise you with a view of the Brighton ski lift just 50 feet below, but this is only a brief distraction and doesn't significantly alter the feeling of remoteness. About half-way up the northern slope of Clayton Peak, the trail turns from a rocky path to a ridge made entirely of rock. For the final stretch leading to the summit, you'll be navigating boulders at a slow pace.

Most Wasatch hikes focus on westward views to the Salt Lake Valley. Clayton Peak offers panoramic views, but the most interesting are those to the east, with Heber Valley in the forefront and the Uintas in the distance.

Photo: Rob Witt

Another view from Clayton Peak

Even near the summit, there are aspens and firs near the trail. At this elevation, snow can cover the ridge into mid-June, and the aspens often change colors in the first week of September. During summer, you may spot deer and coyotes near the ridge, and you'll see chipmunks along the entire trail. Clark's nutcrackers favor the high slopes in the summer, and raptors often circle nearby.

The Great Western Trail is a hike for aspiring peak-baggers, and a good way to train and acclimatize above 10,000 feet. The trail follows the ridgeline, so even when it becomes faint, it's unlikely you'll get too far off-track. From the Clayton Peak summit, you can either return to Guardsman Pass along your ascent route or extend your hike by dropping down to Brighton Lakes or forging on to Sunrise Peak, along the ridge to the southwest.

NEARBY ACTIVITIES

Wasatch Mountain State Park in Midway is just 10 miles down the Guardsman Pass Road to the east. The 22,000-acre park is a year-round mountain retreat with a USGA-sanctioned 27-hole golf course, camping, hiking, and nature trails, and an interpretive center. In winter, snowshoeing and cross-country skiing are popular activities. For reservations or information, call 435-654-1791 or visit **stateparks .utah.gov/parks/wasatch.**

LAKE SOLITUDE
(via the Silver Lake Interpretive Trail)

IN BRIEF

Two hikes for the price of one—the Silver Lake Interpretive Trail circles the alpine marsh around Silver Lake, and the connected Lake Solitude Trail leads through a forest of fir and aspen to a small glacial tarn. You'll get a hands-on education in alpine ecosystems in a scenic mountain setting.

DESCRIPTION

Silver Lake has been one of Salt Lake City's most popular summer recreation areas since July 23, 1849, when more than 2,000 residents escaped the valley's summer heat to hold their first Pioneer Day celebration here. Brighton remains a great summer getaway, and Silver Lake is the ideal short family hike.

Silver Lake, a shallow alpine lake surrounded by wetlands, teems with life during its short season. A brilliantly conceived trail, the Silver Lake Interpretive Trail allows visitors to explore the fragile wetlands ecosystem without ever getting wet or damaging the marshy areas. In the wooded areas along the lake's southern shore, the trail leaves the boardwalk and enters moist woods of fir and aspen along a dirt path.

Start your adventure at the Silver Lake Visitor Center, staffed in summer by the U.S.

Directions

From Salt Lake City's east side, take I-215 south to 6200 South (Exit 6). At the off-ramp, turn left and proceed south 1.7 miles, as 6200 South changes to Wasatch Boulevard (UT 190). Turn left at the signal, staying on UT 190, and continue 14.5 miles up Big Cottonwood Canyon. The Silver Lake Recreation Area and parking are on your right as you enter the Brighton Loop.

KEY AT-A-GLANCE INFORMATION

LENGTH: 3.5 miles round-trip (1 mile on Silver Lake Interpretive Trail, 2.5 miles on Lake Solitude Trail)

ELEVATION GAIN: 500'

ELEVATION AT TRAILHEAD: 8,720'

CONFIGURATION: Loop with out-and-back extension

DIFFICULTY: Easy

SCENERY: Alpine lake with surrounding mountains

EXPOSURE: Partially shaded on Silver Lake Interpretive Trail, mostly shaded on Lake Solitude Trail

TRAFFIC: Busy

TRAIL SURFACE: Boardwalk and dirt

HIKING TIME: 1.5–2 hours

WATER REQUIREMENTS: 1 liter

SEASON: Summer

ACCESS: No fees or permits. Bicycles are prohibited on the Silver Lake boardwalk. The Silver Lake Interpretive Trail is wheelchair-accessible.

MAPS: USGS Brighton

FACILITIES: Restrooms and water at trailhead; store and restaurant across the street. The visitor center is open summer weekends and holidays only, 11 a.m.–5 p.m.

DOGS: Prohibited in Big Cottonwood Canyon, a protected watershed

GPS TRAILHEAD COORDINATES

N40° 36.213´ W111° 35.083´

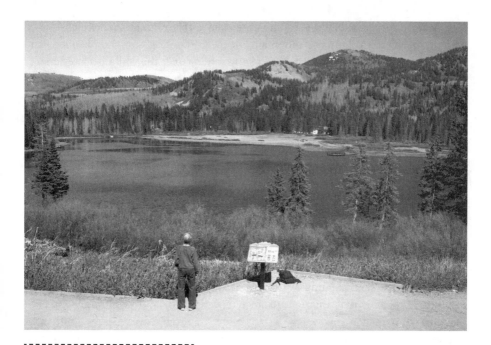

Silver Lake from the interpretive trail

Forest Service. (In winter, the visitor center becomes the Solitude Nordic Center, where cross-country skiers can access 20 kilometers [12 miles] of trails.) From here you can follow the circular path in either direction, although most traffic seems to flow counterclockwise. Along the way, signs and displays describe the area's flora, fauna, and ecosystems, as well as watershed and drinking-water concerns. Rainbow trout and small brook trout stock the lake, making it an ideal destination for young anglers going after their first catch.

Winters are long and life is hard in this alpine environment. With an average of 33 feet of snow each winter, plants and animals have adapted to survive. The quaking aspen photosynthesizes through its bark and doesn't leaf out until mid-June in order to conserve energy. Snowshoe hares turn snow-white in winter and float over the snow with their giant feet. The Uinta ground squirrel, whose burrows line the path, hibernates for eight months of the year.

Wildlife flourishes around the lake and in the wetlands during the summer. Ducks find welcome habitat in the willows, sparrows nest in the nearby trees, and raptors soar overhead. Early-morning visitors may find moose munching on wetland vegetation, while those who arrive later in the day will certainly see their tracks in the boggy marsh. Squirrels start bulking up with seeds and vegetation early in the spring, before returning to their sleep cycle in mid-July.

On the west side of Silver Lake, a wide, well-marked trail leads into woods toward Twin Lakes Reservoir and Lake Solitude. Soon, after crossing a Forest Service road, the trail forks, with the Lake Solitude Trail taking off to the right.

Mature spruce, subalpine fir, and aspen shade the fragrant trail, which is lined with fir needles. Columbine, mountain bluebell, shooting star, monkshood, and other flowers dot the slopes. Patches of snow often cover the trail into late June.

While bikes aren't allowed on the boardwalk, you can expect to see mountain bikers on the Lake Solitude Trail and connecting roads and trails. You'll also pass signs for ski trails, cross ski-resort service roads, and even pass directly under a Solitude ski-resort lift.

Nearing the lake, the trail steepens somewhat but never becomes punishing. Occasionally you'll have to surmount fallen trees, but this only makes the trail more appealing to youngsters. Arriving at the lake, you'll want to explore at least some of the shoreline to the west. Lake Solitude lies at the head of the Mill F South Fork, and you'll cross the stream outlet on the tarn's northwest rim. Mount Evergreen rises above to the south.

As you return to the Silver Lake Interpretive Trail, you'll want to complete the loop and continue your education in alpine ecology. The south shore is more wooded and has several landings that extend into the lake. They are ideal for fishing, but remember that this is a protected watershed, and swimming—or even dangling your feet in the water—is not allowed. From Silver Lake's south side, you can literally watch snowmelt flow into trickles, then into small streams that enter the lake. Within days, you'll be drinking this water at home or in restaurants throughout the valley.

NEARBY ACTIVITIES

Brighton Store and Cafe, across the street from the Silver Lake Visitor Center, provides a convenient stop for a drink, snack, or lunch after your hike (11491 E. Big Cottonwood Canyon Road; 435-649-9156). You can relax at the outdoor eating area and take in the views.

BRIGHTON LAKES (Lake Mary, Lake Martha, Lake Catherine, and Dog Lake)

34

IN BRIEF

Explore a chain of pristine alpine lakes at the top of Big Cottonwood Canyon. It's a favorite hike for families and couples in search of remote mountain scenery, fir-scented woods, and photogenic lakes—all within 30 minutes of your car. Lake Mary may be the most popular alpine hike in the Salt Lake area, with hundreds of hikers enjoying its beauty on any given summer Saturday, but only a small percentage of those hikers go on to Lake Martha or Lake Catherine, where you can often find yourself completely alone. The section from just below Lake Mary to Lake Catherine is part of the Great Western Trail.

DESCRIPTION

Silver mining brought William Stuart Brighton to the upper bowl of Big Cottonwood Canyon in the 1870s. But he soon realized that a better living could be made feeding and housing miners than in actually mining silver.

After spending three summers in a tent, he built a hotel in 1874 near the shores of Silver Lake and soon developed the area into a popular mountain resort. His wife, Catherine, would serve the trout she had caught in Silver Lake with hot buttermilk biscuits.

Directions

From Salt Lake City's east side, take I-215 south to 6200 South (Exit 6). At the off-ramp, turn left and proceed south 1.7 miles, as 6200 South changes to Wasatch Boulevard (UT 190). Turn left at the signal, staying on UT 190, and continue 14.5 miles up Big Cottonwood Canyon. The trailhead is on the southeast side of the Brighton Loop, at the base of the Majestic lift at the Brighton ski resort.

KEY AT-A-GLANCE INFORMATION

LENGTH: 2.2 miles round-trip to Lake Mary + 0.6 miles round-trip to Lake Martha + 1.4 miles round-trip to Lake Catherine + 0.3 mile round-trip to Dog Lake. Total mileage to visit all four lakes is 4.5 miles round-trip.

ELEVATION GAIN: 760' to Lake Mary, 1,200' to Lake Catherine

ELEVATION AT TRAILHEAD: 8,762'

CONFIGURATION: Out-and-back

DIFFICULTY: Moderate

SCENERY: Conifer woods, alpine lakes, glacial cirque

EXPOSURE: Partially shaded

TRAFFIC: Busy

TRAIL SURFACE: Dirt, rock

HIKING TIME: 2.5–3.5 hours

WATER REQUIREMENTS: 1–1.5 liters; water from lakes and streams can be purified.

SEASON: Late spring, summer, early fall

ACCESS: No fees or permits

MAPS: USGS Brighton

FACILITIES: Restrooms, water, and public telephone at Silver Lake Visitor Center

DOGS: Prohibited in Big Cottonwood Canyon, a protected watershed

GPS TRAILHEAD COORDINATES

N40° 35.893′ W111° 35.068′

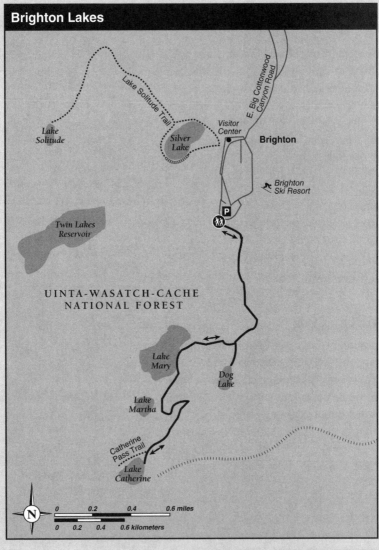

Brighton Lakes

Lake Solitude Trail

E. Big Cottonwood Canyon Road

Lake Solitude

Silver Lake

Visitor Center

Brighton

Brighton Ski Resort

P

Twin Lakes Reservoir

UINTA-WASATCH-CACHE NATIONAL FOREST

Lake Mary

Dog Lake

Lake Martha

Catherine Pass Trail

Lake Catherine

N

| 0 | 0.2 | 0.4 | 0.6 miles |
| 0 | 0.2 | 0.4 | 0.6 kilometers |

10,500 ft.
10,000 ft.
9,500 ft.
9,000 ft.
8,500 ft.
8,000 ft.

Brighton

Lake Mary

Lake Martha

Lake Catherine

0.5 mi.   1 mi.   1.5 mi.   2 mi.   2.2 mi.

Lake Mary, with its granite shore, is a popular family destination.

In winter, Brighton's sons, Will and Dan, made crude skis out of wood just to get around in the deep snow. But skiers would have to wait until 1936 before a towrope was installed to create Brighton, Utah's first ski resort.

Your hike to the beautiful chain of glacial lakes that dot the southern side of Big Cottonwood's upper bowl departs from the base of Brighton Resort's Majestic chairlift. A large sign in front of the lift (at the parking lot's southeast edge) displays the route, marked as the Lake Mary–Catherine Pass Trail.

The trail is steep as it passes beneath two chairlifts and ascends some of Brighton's ski slopes. At 0.6 mile, the trail leaves the slopes and enters a wooded area, offering more of a wilderness feel. At 0.9 mile you come to a gateway of gray granite that forms the bowl of Lake Mary. A large sign at a trail junction marks the spur that leads to Dog Lake. Within moments, a concrete dam—which enlarges and regulates Lake Mary—appears in front of you on the trail. At this point, note an unmarked trail leading off to the right about 30 feet before the dam. It accesses Lake Mary's western side and also leads to Twin Lakes.

The trail ascends to the left of the dam, and within minutes you'll find yourself in the exquisite granite basin that contains Lake Mary. The one-way distance from the trailhead to the Lake Mary shore is 1.1 miles. Even if your ultimate destination is Lake Catherine, you'll want to stop to enjoy the beauty of Lake Mary's granite shoreline. It offers lots of coves, nooks, and smooth granite outcrops where you can pause for a snack and enjoy the view.

The trail continues along Lake Mary's eastern shore for 0.3 mile before arriving at Lake Martha, at an elevation just 38 feet higher than Lake Mary. Lake Martha lacks Lake Mary's granite lining but is perfectly charming and provides more solitude.

At this point, Lake Catherine is just 0.7 mile up the trail, so it would be a shame to miss it. Departing Lake Martha, the crowds thin considerably and the trail, now part of the Great Western Trail, becomes more moist and wooded. Your chances of seeing wildlife—especially moose, deer, and porcupine—increase.

Continuing upward, the trail ascends to the east of Lake Martha, then switches back to the north and comes to a ridgeline promontory overlooking the upper bowl of Big Cottonwood Canyon. The trail continues 0.6 mile past Lake Martha, through alpine forests of spruce and fir, before coming to a crest and a fork in the trail. To the right is the Catherine Pass Trail, which leads over the rim of the cirque into Little Cottonwood Canyon. To the left, the trail arrives at the shore of Lake Catherine in less than 0.1 mile.

In a fitting tribute, William Brighton named the jewel of upper Big Cottonwood Canyon after his wife. Lake Catherine is a perfectly inviting place for a picnic, a rest, or a relaxing afternoon of fishing. Be sure to walk to the top of the granite formation at the north end of the lake, where you'll find the ideal overview of Lake Martha and Lake Mary. On your return trip, Dog Lake is just 700 feet off the main trail below Lake Mary. Although less scenic than the other lakes, it's a great place to watch for moose, particularly in the early morning.

NEARBY ACTIVITIES

Big Cottonwood Canyon provides a field course in Wasatch geology. As you drive up the canyon, a series of large blue-and-brown signs at roadside turnouts provides interpretive information about the canyon. Explaining specific features like folding, faulting, and glaciation, these signs will enrich your hiking experience and give you a better appreciation for the canyon.

SUNSET PEAK 35

IN BRIEF

Sunset Peak is one of the most popular summit trails in the Wasatch. It's a great jaunt, suitable for hikers of all skill levels. Wildlife, wildflowers, and rewarding views along the trail and at the summit justify its popularity.

DESCRIPTION

With a high-elevation trailhead at the top of Little Cottonwood Canyon, a hike from Albion Basin to Catherine Pass offers a chance for nearly any hiker, regardless of skill level or conditioning, to ascend to a high-mountain ridge near the tree line and gaze down at alpine lakes and off to distant ranges. From the Catherine Pass ridgeline, a short climb on to 10,648-foot Sunset Peak delivers even more expansive views stretching east to the Uintas.

The large trailhead parking area fills quickly on weekends, so either come early or plan to take the free shuttle from the Albion Basin entrance station above Alta. An early arrival will also give you the best chance to spot the moose that browse the verdant meadows.

Directions ————————————————➤

From Salt Lake City, go south on I-15 to 9000 South (Exit 295). Turn left onto 9000 South (UT 209) and proceed east 7.2 miles toward the mouth of Little Cottonwood Canyon. Along the way, UT 209 changes names from 9000 South to 9400 South and eventually becomes Little Cottonwood Road. At the mouth of Little Cottonwood Canyon, UT 209 comes to a junction with UT 210. Turn right onto UT 210 and continue 10 miles up Little Cottonwood Canyon to the Albion Basin entrance booth and gate above Alta. Continue 2 miles on the dirt road to the Catherine Pass trailhead parking area, on the right.

KEY AT-A-GLANCE INFORMATION

LENGTH: 4.2 miles round-trip

ELEVATION GAIN: 1,269'

ELEVATION AT TRAILHEAD: 9,379'

CONFIGURATION: Out-and-back

DIFFICULTY: Easy

SCENERY: Wildflowers, alpine scenery, panoramic views from summit

EXPOSURE: Partially shaded

TRAFFIC: Busy

TRAIL SURFACE: Dirt, rock

HIKING TIME: 2–3 hours

WATER REQUIREMENTS: 1 liter; no water at trailhead or on trail

SEASON: Summer

ACCESS: No fees or permits

MAPS: USGS Brighton, Trails Illustrated Wasatch Front (709)

FACILITIES: Restrooms in trailhead parking lot

DOGS: Little Cottonwood Canyon, a protected watershed, prohibits pets and horses.

SPECIAL COMMENTS: The Albion Basin gate above Alta is generally open July 1–November 1.

GPS TRAILHEAD COORDINATES

N40° 34.967´ W111° 37.107´

Bull moose in Albion Basin

Photo: Roy Breslawski/iStockPhoto.com

From the trailhead parking area just south of an Alta chairlift, cross the U.S. Forest Service road and follow the marked trail leading up to Catherine Pass. At 0.2 mile the trail comes to a ski-resort utility road. Turn left onto the road and follow it up and to the left. Leaving the road, the trail soon crosses a granite outcrop and then ascends to the right.

At 0.5 mile, the trail traverses a small wooden bridge and then narrows. It quickly crests at an outcrop, then dips a bit before continuing its ascent. At 0.7 mile, a spur trail leads off to the right to give hikers a nice overview of the Albion Basin, with views of Baldy, Sugarloaf, and Devil's Castle to the left.

Albion Basin is famous for its variety and density of wildflowers. With more than 50 feet of snow per year and a short growing season, the basin is home to dwarf species that have adapted to the harsh environment. An example is alpine asters, with blooms about half the size of the normal species. Both golden and bald eagles can be seen riding the updrafts that rise from the basin to the ridgeline.

At 0.9 mile the trail ascends into a draw with gentle slopes on both sides before entering a small basin meadow. At the upper (east) end of the meadow, the trail climbs a few switchbacks dotted with granite boulders as it makes its way up to Catherine Pass. At Catherine Pass, the trail merges with the Great Western Trail and ascends to the right along a fine, sandy surface leading to Sunset Pass to the south. Here the Great Western Trail continues along the ridge to the south, while the trail to Sunset Peak turns left and to the east. This ridge forms the boundary of Salt Lake and Utah counties.

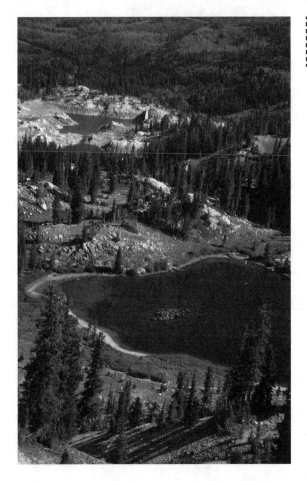

Brighton Lakes (with Lake
Catherine in the foreground),
viewed from Sunset Peak

The trail maintains a steady ascent along a timberline route dotted with subalpine fir. Soon it curves to the left and arrives at the summit. Sunset Peak is the only point in the area to form the boundary of three counties: Salt Lake County to the north and west, Utah County to the south, and Wasatch County to the east. On a clear day you can enjoy excellent views of Mount Timpanogos to the south and Heber Valley to the east. In the distant east, the flat-topped Uintas appear on the horizon. To the north, Lake Catherine is cradled by Mount Tuscarora on the left and Pioneer Peak on the right. Lake Catherine, Lake Martha, and Lake Mary glisten below and almost appear to be adjoining lakes on the same plane.

You can return to the trailhead parking area along your ascent route, or at Sunset Pass take a trail that descends to the west, leading into Albion Basin Campground. From there it's an easy 0.5-mile stroll along the Forest Service road back to the Catherine Pass parking area.

NEARBY ACTIVITIES

The Albion Basin entrance station is a good source of information on hikes and trail conditions in the area. To help reduce automobile traffic, the free Albion Basin Shuttle operates on summer weekends and holidays, 10 a.m.–4:30 p.m. The service offers pickup and drop-off at the entrance station and makes stops at the Catherine Pass trailhead and Albion Basin Campground.

CECRET LAKE 36

IN BRIEF

Albion Basin is ablaze with wildflowers and wildlife in summer. This popular and easy hike travels along a well-marked interpretive trail through flowered meadows to a rock-rimmed alpine lake at the head of Little Cottonwood Canyon.

DESCRIPTION

In its heyday, Alta was a hotbed of silver mining activity. In the 1870s, thirsty miners had 26 saloons to choose from. Many of those miners came from Great Britain and named the area at the head of Little Cottonwood Canyon Albion Basin, evoking an ancient poetic name for their native England.

Today the most valued natural resource in the area is water. Albion Basin receives more than 50 feet of snow per year and provides 15 percent of Salt Lake City's drinking water. Cecret Lake, the small glacial tarn above Albion Basin to the south, serves as the headwaters of Little Cottonwood Creek.

Directions ⟶

From Salt Lake City, go south on I-15 to 9000 South (Exit 295). Turn left onto 9000 South (UT 209) and proceed east 7.2 miles toward the mouth of Little Cottonwood Canyon. Along the way, UT 209 changes names from 9000 South to 9400 South and eventually becomes Little Cottonwood Road. At the mouth of Little Cottonwood Canyon, UT 209 comes to a junction with UT 210. Turn right onto UT 210 and continue 10 miles up Little Cottonwood Canyon to the Albion Basin entrance booth and gate above Alta. Continue 2.5 miles on the dirt road to the Cecret Lake Trailhead parking area, on the left.

KEY AT-A-GLANCE INFORMATION

LENGTH: 1.6 miles round-trip

ELEVATION GAIN: 458'

ELEVATION AT TRAILHEAD: 9,874'

CONFIGURATION: Out-and-back

DIFFICULTY: Easy

SCENERY: Wildflowers, alpine lake, mountain scenery

EXPOSURE: Partially shaded

TRAFFIC: Busy

TRAIL SURFACE: Dirt, rock

HIKING TIME: 1–2 hours

WATER REQUIREMENTS: 1 liter

SEASON: Summer

ACCESS: No fees or permits

MAPS: USGS Brighton, Trails Illustrated Wasatch Front (709)

FACILITIES: Water and restrooms in campground near trailhead

DOGS: Little Cottonwood Canyon, a protected watershed, prohibits pets and horses.

SPECIAL COMMENTS: The gate above Alta is generally open July 1–November 1.

GPS TRAILHEAD COORDINATES

N40° 34.673´ W111° 36.782´

Cecret Lake

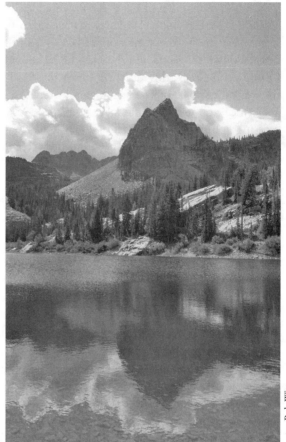

Cecret Lake, with Sundial Peak in the background

Photo: Rob Witt

The other treasured natural resource in the Albion Basin is wildflowers. More than 120 different species bloom in the basin during the short summer season. They start to appear as soon as the snow begins to melt and reach their climax in August. More than 20,000 people come to Albion Basin every summer, so it becomes each visitor's responsibility to tread lightly, stay on the trail, and protect this fragile natural environment.

From the large Cecret Lake parking area, just north of the Albion Basin Campground, take the trail that leads south. It quickly crosses a small brook fed by seasonal runoff from the snow patches that remain well into summer. At 0.1 mile, you'll cross under an Alta ski-resort chairlift before the trail turns onto a dirt road. At 0.2 mile, you'll pass beneath a second Alta chairlift.

At 0.4 mile, the trail leaves the service road and veers to the left. Along the way you'll see several interpretive signs describing the alpine environment and the delicate balance of life that exists in the area. As you pass through this meadow you'll likely see moose grazing on the plant life, especially in the early morning.

At an elevation of 9,500 feet, winters are long and the growing season is short. Wildflowers bloom in a rapid and predictable sequence with sprays of yellow, red, blue, purple, and white. Each color of flower attracts different birds and insects, which then pollinate the flower, enabling it to seed and return the following year. Flies and beetles are drawn to green and brown foliage and flowers, hummingbirds prefer red, and bees will go to any color. As you walk along the main trail, you'll see many side trails leading into the meadow. Most of these work their way back to the campground or the main trail and are always worth exploring.

At 0.6 mile, the trail leaves the flowered basin and crosses a rocky field before ascending a steep slope along a switchback into the upper basin, home to Cecret Lake. Near the northeast side of the lake is a small outlet that allows the water to cascade down the slope and through the meadow below. The headwaters of Little Cottonwood Creek, this outlet continues to be fed by many forks and creeks along the way as it swells to become a raging torrent just 10 miles downstream.

Once you arrive at the lake, you'll see a faint track that circles the shore, crossing boulder fields and talus slopes. Sugarloaf Peak, at 11,051 feet in elevation, lies to the south and can be climbed by scrambling up the slope to the left of the summit.

Moose rarely approach the shores of Cecret Lake, since they find most of their food in the lush lower meadows. But ground squirrels and marmots love the rocky regions near the lake. Because of the lake's popularity, these rodents have become accustomed to humans and are quite fearless. If you leave a pack on the rocks near the lake, you can expect a squirrel to come nosing around looking for a bag of trail mix or crackers.

NEARBY ACTIVITIES

Albion Basin Campground is a perfectly situated base for exploring the upper reaches of Little Cottonwood Canyon. In addition to overnight camping, it's also available for day use, making it an ideal meeting place for families and groups who want to escape the heat in the valley below and spend a day hiking, picnicking, and enjoying the beauty of Albion Basin. Each campsite has a fire grill, parking spur, and picnic table. The campground is open for day use from 7 a.m. to 10 p.m. For reservations, call the National Reservation Service at 877-444-6777 or visit **recreation.gov**.

WHITE PINE LAKE

IN BRIEF

Surprise—a glacial lake in Little Cottonwood Canyon that can be reached along a gently ascending trail. The open trail leads to wonderful canyon views, a glacial cirque dotted with alpine vegetation, and one of the prettiest lakes in Utah.

DESCRIPTION

The loggers and miners who worked Big Cottonwood and Little Cottonwood canyons in the late 1800s and early 1900s were an ambitious lot. They built the first two timber slides in White Pine Canyon and adjoining Red Pine Canyon. Loggers cut Engelmann spruce, which they called white pine, and Douglas-fir, which they called red pine.

After the loggers came miners in search of silver, lead, and zinc. They never made much money, but the miners left their mark in the canyons by building many of the roads to access the mines. The White Pine Trail follows the route of a mining road built in the early 1900s. Don't worry about hiking on jeep trails, though: the U.S. Forest Service closed the road more than 50 years ago, and now it's almost

---

Directions ⟶

From Salt Lake City, go south on I-15 to 9000 South (Exit 295). Turn left onto 9000 South (UT 209) and proceed east 7.2 miles toward the mouth of Little Cottonwood Canyon. Along the way, UT 209 changes names from 9000 South to 9400 South and eventually becomes Little Cottonwood Road. At the mouth of Little Cottonwood Canyon, UT 209 comes to a junction with UT 210. Turn right onto UT 210 and continue 5.2 miles up Little Cottonwood Canyon to the White Pine Trailhead parking lot, on your right.

ℹ KEY AT-A-GLANCE INFORMATION

LENGTH: 9.8 miles round-trip

ELEVATION GAIN: 2,452'

ELEVATION AT TRAILHEAD: 7,698'

CONFIGURATION: Out-and-back

DIFFICULTY: Moderate

SCENERY: Deep glacial valley rising to high glacial lake

EXPOSURE: Mostly shaded to 9,700', partially shaded above 9,700' and at lake

TRAFFIC: Moderate

TRAIL SURFACE: Dirt, rock (mostly rock above 9,800')

HIKING TIME: 5–7 hours

WATER REQUIREMENTS: 1.5–2 liters; springs, streams, and lake provide ample opportunities to purify water.

SEASON: Spring, summer, fall. Ideal snowshoeing or cross-country-skiing trail when snow has stabilized and avalanche risk is minimal.

ACCESS: No fees or permits

MAPS: USGS Dromedary Peak; Trails Illustrated, Uinta National Forest (701), Wasatch Front (709)

FACILITIES: Restrooms at trailhead

DOGS: Little Cottonwood Canyon, a protected watershed, prohibits pets and horses.

GPS TRAILHEAD COORDINATES

N40° 34.537´ W111° 40.868´

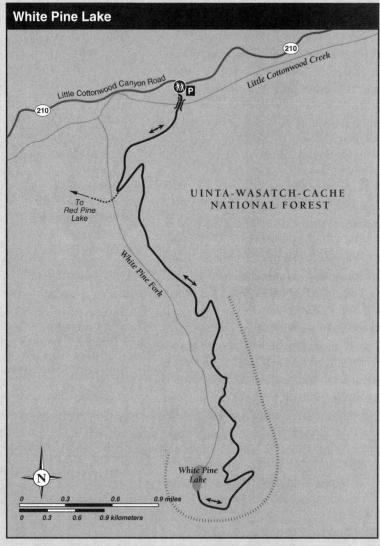

White Pine Lake

210

Little Cottonwood Canyon Road

Little Cottonwood Creek

210

To
Red Pine
Lake

UINTA-WASATCH-CACHE
NATIONAL FOREST

White Pine Fork

N

| 0 | 0.3 | 0.6 | 0.9 miles |
| 0 | 0.3 | 0.6 | 0.9 kilometers |

White Pine
Lake

12,000 ft.
11,000 ft.
10,000 ft.
9,000 ft.
8,000 ft.
7,000 ft.

White Pine
Fork

White Pine
Lake

1 mi.   2 mi.   3 mi.   4 mi.   4.9 mi.

Photo: Rob Witt

White Pine Lake in the late fall

completely reclaimed. It looks and feels like a wide trail, not a rutted jeep trail, allowing you to walk side-by-side with your hiking companion. Its openness reduces the chances of getting lost, so the hike is well suited and safe for inexperienced hikers and children who are capable of the distance. Because the trail began as a road, the gradient is not as steep as most trails', but the route is longer and more circuitous.

The trail departs from the south side of the large White Pine Trailhead parking lot. Even though the parking lot accommodates 35 cars, it often fills on summer weekends, and latecomers may find themselves parking along Little Cottonwood Canyon Road. From the parking area the trail dips, and within 100 yards you cross Little Cottonwood Creek and begin your ascent.

Immediately after crossing the bridge, the trail passes through an area damaged by avalanche. Looking at some of the leveled aspens with trunk diameters in excess of a foot, you get a sense of the power and force of snow thundering down the mountain. The White Pine Trail is a popular snowshoeing and cross-country-skiing area, but only after the avalanche danger has passed.

At 0.9 mile you arrive at a junction with the Red Pine Trail. With the White Pine Fork at your right, continue along the wide trail as it makes a sharp turn to the left and ascends along a straight course. At the top of this stretch you arrive at a canyon overlook at 8,200 feet in elevation before making a hairpin turn and continuing through forests of conifer and aspen.

By now the trail is high above the canyon floor, following a well-crafted path along the eastern side of White Pine Fork. Along the way, numerous springs and creeks cross the trail. Wildflowers, including white columbine and buttercups, dot the side of the trail.

At 3.4 miles the trail enters a large open meadow, and the upper reaches of the glacial bowl become more apparent. Soon the terrain changes from dense spruce and fir forests to a rocky glacial terrain. Near the top of the canyon, the trail crosses a wide talus slope, often covered by a snowfield into early summer. Once you cross the slope, the trail remains on glacial moraine to the rim above the lake. As the trail nears the lake, at an elevation just under 10,000 feet, the trail sweeps widely to the east, then turns west as it rounds the bowl and heads toward the lake. You might think it faster to scramble the slope to the west and drop down directly into White Pine Lake, but even though the trail looks long, you can move quickly along its gradual ascent.

Within minutes you'll be at the rim overlooking White Pine Lake, the high elevation for the hike. From there, a downhill stroll of 0.2 mile will put you at the water's edge. If you're an early riser, you can sit on one of the smooth granite boulders and watch trout jump from the lake to snag live flies. If you look up the drainage to the south, you may see deer grazing on the sparse high grasses. Marmot and pica also find a welcoming habitat in the surrounding boulder fields.

White Pine Lake provides a beautiful setting for a relaxing lunch before you return. By crossing the boulder fields and ridge directly to the west, you can also drop into the Red Pine Lake basin and return to the trailhead from there. This traverse involves some scrambling and navigating your way along an unmarked route before arriving at Red Pine Lake, about 360 feet below White Pine Lake's elevation. This makes for an enjoyable loop hike, but come prepared with a detailed topo map and solid route-finding skills before attempting the traverse.

Note: White Pine Lake is adjacent to the Lone Peak Wilderness Area. Bicycles are permitted on the trail all the way to the lake, although you can expect some rocky terrain.

NEARBY ACTIVITIES

The White Pine Trail offers some spectacular scenery and a beautiful lake, but no major waterfalls. If you yearn to see a canyon stream spraying and cascading over granite cliffs, try **Lisa Falls,** just 2.5 miles down the canyon from the White Pine Trailhead. The Lisa Falls trailhead is on the north side of the road. The path climbs along the stream for 0.1 mile before arriving at the falls.

PFEIFFERHORN
(via Red Pine Lake) 38

IN BRIEF

Pfeifferhorn is one of the best summit hikes in the Wasatch. A scenic canyon trail leads to a glistening alpine lake. A challenging traverse over a saddle of large boulders and a steep scramble to the 11,326-foot summit offer wonderful views.

DESCRIPTION

The Pfeifferhorn (identified as Little Matterhorn Peak on USGS maps) is recognizable from the floor of both Salt Lake Valley and Utah Valley by its distinctive pyramid shape and its location behind Lone Peak, on Little Cottonwood's southern ridge. Lying within the rugged Lone Peak Wilderness Area, the mountain was named in honor of Chuck Pfeiffer, an early leader of the Wasatch Mountain Club.

A climb of the Pfeifferhorn offers hikers an excellent variety of trail scenery, alpine lakes, boulder-hopping, and a challenging scramble to the top. In spite of the challenges, the Pfeifferhorn remains one of the most popular summit climbs in the Wasatch.

From the White Pine trailhead parking lot, the trail descends to the south to cross

KEY AT-A-GLANCE INFORMATION

LENGTH: 7 miles round-trip to Red Pine Lake, 10 miles round-trip to Pfeifferhorn summit

ELEVATION GAIN: 3,628'

ELEVATION AT TRAILHEAD: 7,698'

CONFIGURATION: Out-and-back

DIFFICULTY: Hard

SCENERY: Wooded canyon, alpine lakes, summit views

EXPOSURE: Mostly shaded to Red Pine Lake; partially shaded to saddle; no shade from saddle to summit

TRAFFIC: Moderate

TRAIL SURFACE: Dirt and rock to lake, mostly rock from lake to summit

HIKING TIME: 7–9 hours

WATER REQUIREMENTS: 2–3 liters; water in nearby streams and lakes can be purified.

SEASON: Late spring–early fall

ACCESS: No fees or permits

MAPS: USGS Dromedary Peak

FACILITIES: Restrooms and water at trailhead

DOGS: Little Cottonwood Canyon, a protected watershed, prohibits pets and horses.

Directions

From Salt Lake City, go south on I-15 to 9000 South (Exit 295). Turn left onto 9000 South (UT 209) and proceed east 7.2 miles toward the mouth of Little Cottonwood Canyon. Along the way, UT 209 changes names from 9000 South to 9400 South and eventually becomes Little Cottonwood Road. At the mouth of Little Cottonwood Canyon, UT 209 comes to a junction with UT 210. Turn right onto UT 210 and continue 5.2 miles up Little Cottonwood Canyon to the White Pine trailhead parking lot, on your right.

GPS TRAILHEAD COORDINATES

N40° 34.537´ W111° 40.868´

Pfeifferhorn (via Red Pine Lake)

210

Tanners
Flat

Little Cottonwood Creek

White Pine Fork

LONE PEAK
WILDERNESS

Maybird
Gulch

Red Pine
Dam

Red Pine
Lake

Upper Red
Pine Lake

White Pine
Lake

SALT LAKE COUNTY
UTAH COUNTY

Pfeifferhorn

N

| 0 | 0.3 | 0.6 | 0.9 miles |
| 0 | 0.3 | 0.6 | 0.9 kilometers |

12,000 ft.						Pfeifferhorn Summit
11,000 ft.						
10,000 ft.				Red Pine Lake		
9,000 ft.			Red Pine Fork			
8,000 ft.						
7,000 ft.						
	1 mi.	2 mi.	3 mi.	4 mi.	5 mi.	

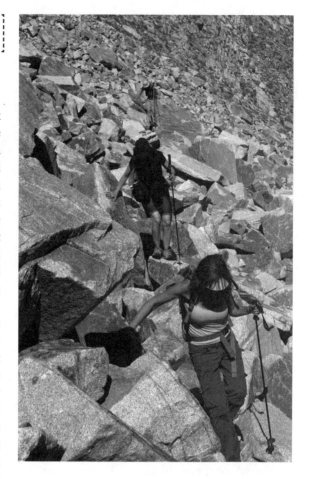

Boulder-hopping on the way to the summit

Little Cottonwood Creek over a wooden bridge. The trail then begins with a steady ascent along an old mining road into the mouth of White Pine Canyon. An early start will give you the best opportunity to spot deer and moose on the trail below Red Pine Lake, and will give you plenty of time to reach the summit.

At 0.8 mile, you arrive at a junction where the mining road ascends to the left on its way to White Pine Lake. Avoid this route by continuing straight ahead for another 20 feet. Here the trail climbs to the left before immediately turning right and crossing a bridge over White Pine Fork. After the bridge crossing, the trail ascends to the northwest as it makes its way around the canyon wall to enter Red Pine Canyon. As the trail moves up into the canyon, you'll have a fleeting glimpse of the Pfeifferhorn to the south.

At 2.1 miles from the trailhead, you'll arrive at a steep stretch littered with boulders and marked by avalanche scarring. Soon the trail unites with Red Pine Creek and levels out a bit. At 2.5 miles you'll pass the cutoff and bridge to Maybird Gulch, on your right. Immediately after the cutoff, the trail passes through a boggy meadow where the stream spills onto the trail and passes mine tailings on the left. A steep, rocky section of trail brings you to the shores of Red Pine Lake. With a steady pace, you can hike from the trailhead to the lake in just under 2 hours.

Once on the north shore of Red Pine Lake, take a moment to enjoy the view and plan your route to the summit. The Pfeifferhorn is not visible from Red Pine Lake, but it lies to the southwest, obscured by the rocky slopes to the west of the lake. The easiest, most reliable route to the summit starts by following the trail along the east side of the lake. Although it may look more direct and very appealing, avoid the talus field to the west of the lake.

Arriving at the south end of the lake, you pass a large rock slab the size of a school bus on your right. Cross the creek that descends from Upper Red Pine Lake and climb a beautiful section of steep trail leading through fragrant stands of spruce. This trail winds its way up and to the southwest, eventually rising above the wooded area onto a steep, rocky slope leading toward the saddle.

The most impressive feature of the climb from Red Pine Lake to the Pfeifferhorn summit is the quality of the rock. Often mistaken for granite, the talus slopes, saddle, and summit of the Pfeifferhorn are composed almost entirely of quartz monzonite, an intrusive igneous rock. Quartz monzonite provides an excellent climbing and nonskid hiking surface, making boulder-hopping on the route a true delight.

Once at the saddle, you'll have a clear view of the Pfeifferhorn down the ridgeline to the west. But before ascending the final 500 feet to the summit, you need to traverse a 100-yard-long, knife-edged, boulder-capped saddle. Although no technical-climbing equipment is necessary, navigation does require moving carefully over and around large boulders with some exposure. You'll want to stow your trekking poles in your pack and consider bringing along a pair of gloves to protect your hands. Most hikers pick a route that stays primarily to the right or north side of the ridge.

Once off the boulders, the trail resumes its steep climb up a chute to the left of the peak's southeast ridge. From the massive slabs that form the small summit platform, you'll have great views into the populated valleys. The most intriguing views, though, are those directly below as you survey the wild, rocky, and rugged terrain of the Lone Peak Wilderness. From the Pfeifferhorn summit, you'll find some challenging descent routes into Maybird Gulch and Bells Canyon to the north and west, but most day hikers are content with a return to Red Pine Lake and back to Little Cottonwood Canyon.

Note: Little Cottonwood Canyon may have avalanche closures November 1–May 15.

NEARBY ACTIVITIES

The brilliant quartz monzonite that graces the summit of both Pfeifferhorn and Lone Peak was also admired by early Mormon pioneers, who quarried the stone for the building of the Salt Lake Temple. The **Temple Quarry Trail** is a 0.3-mile, wheelchair-accessible interpretive loop trail that will give you a greater appreciation for the monumental effort involved in quarrying stone. The trailhead is at the mouth of Little Cottonwood Canyon on UT 209 just south of its intersection with UT 210, the main canyon road.

AMERICAN FORK TWIN PEAKS 39

IN BRIEF

This challenging route along a knife ridge and up a steep rocky slope leads to the dual summit that forms the highest peak in Salt Lake County. In just over a mile one-way, you'll achieve a first-class mountaineering scramble capped by commanding views in all directions.

DESCRIPTION

Let's begin with a pop quiz: What is the most frequently summited 11,000-plus-foot peak in Utah?

If you guessed Mount Timpanogos or even Kings Peak, you're thinking clearly, but neither of those peaks come close to the hundreds of skiers and summer visitors who reach the summit of 11,000-foot Hidden Peak at the top of Snowbird's Aerial Tram. The highest lift-accessed peak in the Wasatch, Hidden Peak is also a convenient trailhead for climbing American Fork Twin Peaks along the ridge to the southwest. In spite of the crowds that ride the tram to the top of Hidden Peak, very few ever make the traverse to the summit of Twin Peaks. You might enjoy the entire route to yourself, even on a summer weekend.

Directions

From Salt Lake City, go south on I-15 to 9000 South (Exit 295). Turn left onto 9000 South (UT 209) and proceed 7.2 miles east toward the mouth of Little Cottonwood Canyon. Along the way, UT 209 changes names from 9000 South to 9400 South and eventually becomes Little Cottonwood Road. At the mouth of Little Cottonwood Canyon, UT 209 comes to a junction with UT 210. Turn right onto UT 210 and continue 8 miles up Little Cottonwood Canyon to the Snowbird parking area, on your right. The tram base is in the Snowbird Center, on the Plaza Deck.

KEY AT-A-GLANCE INFORMATION

LENGTH: 2.2 miles round-trip

ELEVATION GAIN: 660' (from top of Snowbird Aerial Tram)

ELEVATION AT TRAILHEAD: 11,000' (summit of Hidden Peak, at top of tram)

CONFIGURATION: Out-and-back

DIFFICULTY: Moderate

SCENERY: High-alpine rock slopes and spectacular views

EXPOSURE: No shade on trail

TRAFFIC: Light

TRAIL SURFACE: Dirt, rock

HIKING TIME: 2.5–3 hours

WATER REQUIREMENTS: 1–1.5 liters

SEASON: Late spring, summer, early fall

ACCESS: Hike lies on U.S. Forest Service land accessed through Snowbird Resort. You must buy a ticket to ride the aerial tram to the Hidden Peak summit (see page 176 for prices).

MAPS: USGS Dromedary Peak, Trails Illustrated Wasatch Front (709)

FACILITIES: Restrooms and water at Hidden Peak trailhead

DOGS: Little Cottonwood Canyon, a protected watershed, prohibits pets and horses.

SPECIAL COMMENTS: You can also climb Twin Peaks unassisted from Snowbird's Gad Valley.

GPS TRAILHEAD COORDINATES

N40° 33.640´ W111° 38.727´

Photo: Michael Madsen/iStockPhoto.com

East and West Twin Peaks, viewed from Snowbird's Hidden Peak

American Fork Twin Peaks lies across the canyon and to the east of Broads Fork (or Salt Lake) Twin Peaks. The East Twin is 11,433 feet and the West Twin is 11,489 feet, making the West Twin the highest peak in Salt Lake County. The ridge-line constitutes the county line, with Utah County lying to the south. The scramble from Hidden Peak to Twin Peaks is one of the more challenging sections of a longer hike from Albion Basin to Red Pine Lake known as the Bullion Divide.

The Snowbird Aerial Tram achieves 2,900 feet of vertical lift in about 1.6 miles. From the top of the tram, walk down the road to the southwest that leads into Mineral Basin. About 0.1 mile down the road, the rocky thumb of a ridge forms to the west. Ascend the ridge along a faint trail as it becomes rockier and more jag-ged. An occasional subalpine fir or limber pine will dot the ridgeline's rocks, but for the most part the route is treeless, even as it dips below the 11,000-foot tree line.

As the knife ridge dips down to an elevation of about 10,800 feet, you'll encounter the most challenging sections of the trail, with some exposure and long sections that require the use of both hands and some basic climbing moves. Along the way you may be tempted to take a lower route, but you'll find that the ridgeline rocks are large and stable, while the rocks just 8–10 feet below the ridge are small and loose.

As you near the end of the ridgeline scramble, a formation of black rock leads up toward the eastern slope of East Twin. Follow this dike while still staying close to the top of the ridge. Use extreme caution: the black rock has particularly sharp edges. Even the slightest fall could result in severe injury.

The 100-yard ascent from the knife ridge to the summit of East Twin follows a faint but discernible trail that zigzags up the steep, rocky slope. You'll often spot mountain goats grazing on these slopes. From the bald, rounded summit of East Twin, it's a leisurely 10-minute stroll along rocky tundra to the West Twin summit. Another route from East Twin leads to a little-known and rarely visited South Twin, at the end of a gentle tundra ridge 0.3 mile to the south. Most summer days will be clear and refreshing at the summit, but don't come if storm clouds form: with any chance of lightning, Twin Peaks' exposed ridge and expansive summit is the last place you want to be.

You'll find exceptional views in all directions. Some of the highlights include the back side of Mount Timpanogos, Heber Valley to the east, and the many peaks along the Little Cottonwood and Big Cottonwood ridgelines. From the summit, descend one of the steep couloirs to the north into Gad Valley or return along the ridge back to the tram at Hidden Peak.

Note: Prices to ride the Snowbird Aerial Tram are as follows: single ride, $16 adults, $14 ages 7–16 and seniors 65 and older, free for children age 6 and younger; all-day access, $22 adults, $18 ages 7–16 and seniors 65 and older, free for children age 6 and younger.

NEARBY ACTIVITIES

Snowbird offers a varied selection of summer activities for all ages and interests. Whether you rent bikes and mountain scooters or bring your own, you can ride on easier trails near the base or on the expert trails that descend from the top of the tram. ATV and horseback riding tours are available in Mineral Basin. Other choices: spend the day riding the alpine slide, zipline, and mechanical bull or doing acrobatics on the bungee trampoline, then visit the Cliff Spa to recover. You'll also find restaurants, shopping, and accommodations on-site. For a schedule of events, concerts, classes, and activities, visit **snowbird.com**.

BELLS CANYON

IN BRIEF

Bells Canyon is a long, deep, beautiful canyon with cascading falls, lush vegetation, and a rocky cirque. The trail is steep and challenging, but the varied views and granite setting are spectacular.

DESCRIPTION

Rising from the valley floor to a high glacial bowl below the summit of Lone Peak, Bells Canyon is as appealing to geologists as it is to hikers. Because the glacier that formed this canyon reached the foot of the mountains and the elevation of Lake Bonneville, Bells Canyon is geologically unique. This allows geologists to study glacial advance and the lake's rising elevation. Equally fascinating are the exposed Precambrian rocks at the mouth of Bells Canyon, some of the oldest rocks on earth.

Immediately south of Little Cottonwood Canyon, within the federally protected Lone Peak Wilderness Area, Bells Canyon is easily accessible from a low-elevation suburban trailhead. From the parking area, the trail makes a steep switchback ascent onto the moraine of the glacier that once filled the canyon.

After 0.7 mile of sage-and-oak-covered foothills, you'll come to a dirt utility road

KEY AT-A-GLANCE INFORMATION

LENGTH: 5.6 miles round-trip to upper waterfall, 8.4 miles round-trip to Upper Bells Canyon Reservoir

ELEVATION GAIN: 2,361' to upper waterfall, 4,149' to Upper Bells Canyon Reservoir

ELEVATION AT TRAILHEAD: 5,239'

CONFIGURATION: Out-and-back

DIFFICULTY: Hard

SCENERY: Deep wooded canyon, waterfalls, towering canyon walls, some valley views

EXPOSURE: Mostly shaded

TRAFFIC: Light

TRAIL SURFACE: Dirt, rock

HIKING TIME: 2.5–3 hours to upper waterfall, 6–8 hours to Upper Bells Canyon Reservoir

WATER REQUIREMENTS: 2–3 liters; water in stream and reservoir can be purified.

SEASON: Spring, summer, fall

ACCESS: No fees or permits

MAPS: USGS Draper; Trails Illustrated Wasatch Front (709), Uinta National Forest (701)

FACILITIES: Restrooms and water at trailhead

DOGS: Prohibited in Bells Canyon, a protected watershed

Directions

From Salt Lake City, go south on I-15 to 9000 South (Exit 295). Turn left onto 9000 South (UT 209) and proceed east 6.1 miles toward the mouth of Little Cottonwood Canyon. Along the way, UT 209 changes names from 9000 South to 9400 South and eventually becomes East Little Cottonwood Road. The Granite trailhead, which provides access to Bells Canyon and other local trails, is at 3470 E. Little Cottonwood Road.

GPS TRAILHEAD COORDINATES

N40° 34.305′ W111° 47.813′

Bells Canyon

Steep canyon walls and valley views from Bells Canyon Trail

leading up toward the mouth of the canyon. The shallow waters of the drained Lower Bells Canyon Reservoir are on the right. You can frequently see such migrating waterfowl as ducks and Canada geese around the pondlike remains of the reservoir, and deer on the slopes above it.

After 100 yards on the utility road, take an unmarked trail that leads off to the left. This trail ascends gently at first through bigtooth maple and curly-leaf mountain mahogany. At 1.3 miles from the trailhead, the path crosses a sturdy wooden footbridge to the south side of a stream.

The trail enters the mouth of Bells Canyon along a granite-strewn pathway that is sometimes overgrown but easy to follow. As you ascend the canyon, conifers become more predominant and aspens begin to appear. Along the way, several spur trails depart from the main trail, but stay on the main trail, defined by the granite boulders. At about 1.7 miles from the trailhead, you'll come to a junction with a spur trail leading off to the left. A steep descent on this spur takes you to the base of the lower falls. You may want to make this the destination for a short day hike.

From the lower falls, the main trail continues its vertical ascent along a staircase of granite boulders. After 2.2 miles from the trailhead, the steps ease up a bit, but the dirt trail is still punctuated with plenty of granite.

At 2.6 miles, the trail meets with the stream on the left and a large granite slab on the right. Follow the trail across the slab, and within a few minutes you'll arrive at the smaller upper falls. This is a great destination in its own right and certainly

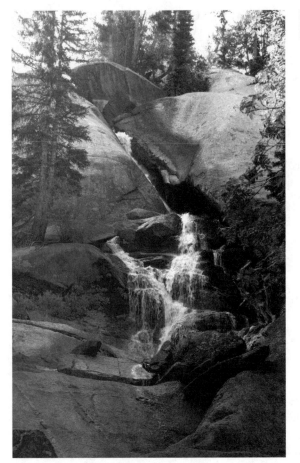

Bells Canyon waterfall

worth a rest stop and trail snack. At this elevation the forest is dense and moist; ferns and moss line the trail, and spruce and aspen provide the canopy.

To continue upward, look for a crude log bridge 100 feet below the waterfall. The bridge crosses the stream to the north side of the creek. This trail leads initially through a dense passage of fern before it ascends a granite slope. The trail passes through a meadow and then crosses the creek over another log bridge on its way to the Upper Bells Canyon Reservoir.

Within a rocky cirque, the upper reservoir is a remote, pristine glacial lake at an elevation of 9,388 feet. The reservoir is surrounded by Lone Peak, Bearstooth, and Thunder Mountain. Any routes leading beyond the reservoir in the direction of those peaks require difficult scrambling and technical climbing expertise. The most reliable way out of the canyon is to retrace your route and descend the steep granite stairs back to the trailhead.

NEARBY ACTIVITIES

The **Rocky Mouth Canyon Trail** is a short, scenic hike through a slot canyon to a beautiful waterfall. The trailhead is at 11300 S. Wasatch Blvd. in Sandy. (Be sure to park at the trailhead and not in the neighborhood.) The first 0.25 mile follows a sidewalk to a dirt trail, which continues another 0.25 mile to the waterfall.

LONE PEAK
(via Jacobs Ladder)

IN BRIEF

The toughest, and perhaps the most reward-ing, of these 60 hikes. A Lone Peak ascent demands a long, dry, steep approach into a beautiful rock bowl surrounded by towering cliffs. The final climb to the summit over mas-sive rock slabs offers spectacular views.

DESCRIPTION

Lone Peak is the prominent summit that dominates both the south end of the Salt Lake Valley and the north end of Utah Valley. Its west-lying ridge trails off into the valley at Point of the Mountain. The jagged spires and sheer rock face of the 11,253-foot summit are identifiable from miles around. But only those who hike into the Lone Peak Wilderness Area and approach the mountain's higher reaches can appreciate the impressive and inspiring qualities of Lone Peak.

While many routes lead to the summit of Lone Peak, all are difficult and require 5,000–6,000 feet of vertical elevation gain. Population

----

Directions ⟶

From Salt Lake City, go south on I-15 to 12300 South (Exit 291). Turn left and proceed east 1.9 miles on 12300 South (UT 71) to 1300 East. Turn right and drive south 0.2 mile on 1300 East to the traffic circle. Enter the traffic circle and make a three-quarter loop, exiting east-bound onto Pioneer Road. Continue east 1 mile on Pioneer Road to 2000 East. Turn right on 2000 East and continue south 0.2 mile to the Orson Smith trailhead, at 12601 S. 2000 East. From the Orson Smith trailhead parking area, turn right on Upper Corner Canyon Road, a dirt road that leads south. Continue 2.6 miles on Upper Corner Canyon Road to the Ghost Falls trailhead parking area.

KEY AT-A-GLANCE INFORMATION

LENGTH: 12 miles round-trip
ELEVATION GAIN: 5,460'
ELEVATION AT TRAILHEAD: 5,793'
CONFIGURATION: Out-and-back
DIFFICULTY: Hard
SCENERY: Rocky high-alpine basins, rock cliffs, exceptional summit views
EXPOSURE: Partial shade in lower bowl between 9,200' and 10,000'. Remainder of trail is fully exposed. Dry, exposed, south-facing slopes can be particularly hot in the summer.
TRAFFIC: Moderate
TRAIL SURFACE: Dirt, rock
HIKING TIME: 8–11 hours
WATER REQUIREMENTS: 3–4 liters; no water on trail after spring snowmelt
SEASON: Late spring, summer, and early fall
ACCESS: No fees or permits. Corner Canyon Road is open 6 a.m.–10 p.m. up to the Ghost Falls trailhead.
MAPS: USGS Draper; Trails Illustrated Uinta National Forest (701)
FACILITIES: No restrooms or water at trailhead
DOGS: The long distance, lack of water, and exposed rock-scrambling to the summit make this hike unsuit-able for them.

GPS TRAILHEAD COORDINATES

N40° 29.655´ W111° 49.002´

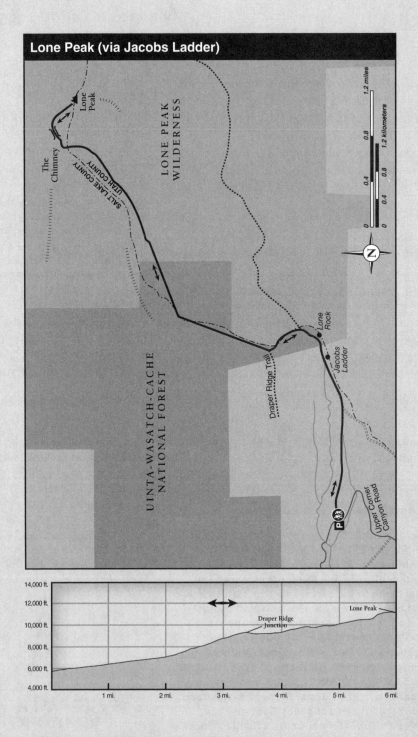

Lone Peak (via Jacobs Ladder)

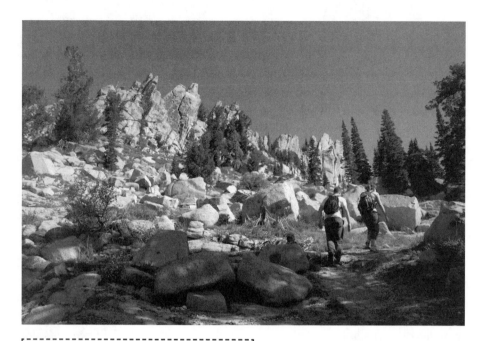

Ascending through boulders to the Lone Peak cirque

growth in Draper, where residential subdivisions abut national forest, has diminished access to some trails. The Jacobs Ladder Trail, starting at the Ghost Falls trailhead, has emerged in recent years as one of the more popular and accessible summit routes. Like other Lone Peak trails, Jacobs Ladder, leading to the Draper Ridge, is long, dry, and steep.

From the trailhead parking area, continue up the road another 50 yards to an opening in the fence on your left. Take this singletrack mountain-bike trail as it winds through scrubby woods to a low-lying ridgeline. The unmarked trail follows this ridge in an easterly direction as it parallels, merges, and diverges from various bike tracks. In less than 1 mile, the trail approaches a chalky white outcrop and curves north along a much narrower trail to begin the Jacobs Ladder climb. It's a steep ascent through Gambel oak, sage, and curly-leaf mountain mahogany, leading up to Draper Ridge.

At 3.3 miles, the Jacobs Ladder Trail meets the Draper Ridge Trail on a dry slope at an elevation of 9,120 feet. At this point you've been climbing for about 2 hours and you've gained more than 3,300 feet, or about two-thirds of your overall vertical ascent for the hike. Take a short rest on the nearby log and know that the toughest part of the trail is behind you—and the most beautiful section is right in front of you.

From the Draper Ridge junction, the trail descends slightly into a meadow dotted with quartz monzonite and lined with conifers. As it rises above the meadow, the trail crosses giant slabs of rock, appropriately marked by cairns. From the meadow to the summit, the trail surface is predominately rock, dotted with spruce and fir, then alpine tundra nearing the tree line. Crossing exposed slabs before entering a narrow, boulder-strewn draw, the trail leads to the upper cirque. Along this rock route it's easy to lose the trail, but as long as you maintain an ascent in a northeasterly direction toward the upper cirque, you're on track.

Arriving at the cirque, you'll be awestruck by the full view of Lone Peak's summit cliffs on the right. As you stand in the cirque facing due north, the cliffs will be at the 3 o'clock position. Either follow the cairns or walk up toward the boxy chute at 1 o'clock. Some easy Class 3 scrambling will lead you up the chute, known as The Chimney.

As you emerge from The Chimney on the west side of the ridge, the trail crosses over the ridge and follows a faint route up a rocky slope to the large boulders that compose the summit formation. As you make your final approach to the summit, cautiously weaving your way through the massive angular slabs, it's hard to ignore the stunning majesty of the peak and cliffs in front of you. Lone Peak is one of the most breathtakingly beautiful summits in the United States.

The summit block of Lone Peak has enough space for just a few climbers to sit and enjoy the views. Lone Peak is not the highest peak in the Wasatch—it's not even the highest peak in the Lone Peak Wilderness Area—but it does have the most commanding views. Because of its forefront position, Lone Peak is one summit from which you have unobstructed views of every other major peak in the Wasatch, as well as extended views to the north and south. Take time to enjoy these views before beginning your long, dry descent back to the trailhead.

Note: Horses, bicycles, motorized vehicles, and open campfires are prohibited in the Lone Peak Wilderness Area.

NEARBY ACTIVITIES

The **Orson Smith trailhead** (12601 S. 2000 East) provides a convenient and well-maintained starting point for many area hikes. The park has restrooms, water, picnic tables, and signs showing the area's trail system. From the trailhead you can access the Bonneville Shoreline Trail, the Aqueduct Trail, the Orson Smith Trail, and other connector trails. You can also reach two Lone Peak trails—Little Willow Trail and Cherry Canyon Trail—from the Orson Smith trailhead.

YELLOW FORK

IN BRIEF

A multiuse trail in the Oquirrh Mountain foothills of Rose Canyon gives hikers, bikers, and horseback riders easy access to some gentle canyon trails and less-familiar views of the Salt Lake Valley.

DESCRIPTION

The southwest side of the Salt Lake Valley has a history of ranching and mining going back to 1848—just months after Mormon pioneers arrived—when brothers Sanford and Thomas Bingham discovered copper ore in the canyon where they grazed cattle and horses. When they advised Brigham Young of their find, he discouraged them from staking a claim since the primary concern of the fledgling colony was survival and establishing settlements. Following Young's counsel, the Bingham brothers left their name on the canyon but relinquished mining rights to others, who in 1863 began digging what would eventually become the world's deepest open-pit mine (see Nearby Activities).

In this corner of the Salt Lake Valley, mining camps and cattle rustling were a part of the fabric of everyday life into the 1920s. It seems that recreation and culture never really

KEY AT-A-GLANCE INFORMATION

LENGTH: 5 miles round-trip (to knoll and back)

ELEVATION GAIN: 725'

ELEVATION AT TRAILHEAD: 5,648'

CONFIGURATION: Out-and-back, with various side-canyon routes and optional loops

DIFFICULTY: Easy

SCENERY: Canyon and valley views

EXPOSURE: Partially shaded

TRAFFIC: Light

TRAIL SURFACE: Dirt, rock

HIKING TIME: 2.5–3.5 hours

WATER REQUIREMENTS: 1–2 liters

SEASON: Spring, summer, fall; snowshoeing in winter

ACCESS: No fees or permits. The trail lies within Yellow Fork Canyon County Park.

MAPS: USGS Tickville Spring

FACILITIES: No restrooms or water at trailhead

DOGS: On leash

Directions

From Draper, take I-15 south to the Bangerter Highway/UT 154 turnoff (Exit 289) and head west. Continue 5.2 miles to the traffic signal at 134th South and turn left. Go west 3.2 miles on 134th South to Rose Canyon Road (6400 West) and turn left. Continue 0.6 mile to the stop sign and turn right. Continue another 3.5 miles on Rose Canyon Road, through a rural area with ranches and horse lots, before arriving at a small trailhead-parking area.

GPS TRAILHEAD COORDINATES

N40° 27.920´ W112° 5.088´

Yellow Fork

Dry Canyon

Shaggy Mountain Road

Rose Canyon

Yellow Fork Canyon Road

YELLOW FORK
CANYON COUNTY
PARK

Yellow Fork

Rose Canyon Road

Arnold Hollow Road

Step Mountain Road

Water Fork

knoll

N

0   0.2   0.4   0.6 miles

0   0.2   0.4   0.6 kilometers

CAMP WILLIAM
MILITARY RESERVATION

7,000 ft.

6,500 ft.   Knoll

6,000 ft.
        Side Canyon

5,500 ft.

5,000 ft.

4,500 ft.

        0.5 mi.   1 mi.   1.5 mi.   2 mi.   2.5 mi.

Horseback riders at the mouth of Yellow Fork

gained much of a foothold in this rural blue-collar area—those were reserved for the Cottonwood Canyons or downtown, not for Herriman or Copperton, where folks had work to do.

As the population of Salt Lake County grew, development stretched south, and in 1999 Herriman City was incorporated, quickly becoming one of the fastest-growing master-planned communities in Utah. Because a youthful and growing population needs recreation areas, ranchers and miners in the nearby canyons in the foothills of the Oquirrh Mountains are getting accustomed to sharing resources with mountain bikers and hikers.

As you stand in the trailhead parking area, you'll see two small spring-fed trickles of water that merge before you to flow into Rose Canyon—although considering their minuscule size, they aren't exactly carving the canyon. To the left is Water Fork, which has its source at Rose Canyon Spring, 2 miles up the canyon to the southwest. To the right is Yellow Fork, which is fed by at least two springs up the canyon to the northwest. You'll be ascending along Yellow Fork by following the trail—an old ranching and mining road—past the gate on your right.

Depending on the season, you may see hikers, bikers, horse riders, or snowshoers on the trail—all are welcome in this multiuse county park. If walking on the dirt road isn't your preference, you'll find numerous narrow hiking trails that parallel the creek and offer a bit more solitude and shade.

As you ascend into the gentle terrain and peaceful solitude of Yellow Fork, it's easy to transport yourself back to the 1850s and imagine exploring this canyon for the first time. You hear a rustle in the undergrowth and make a quick turn to see a wild turkey take flight. You wonder if a coyote, or perhaps even a cougar, is watching you from the rocky ridgeline just a few hundred yards to the left. You'll pass mature juniper trees and bigtooth maples, and the Gambel oaks are some of the largest and oldest such trees in Utah.

At 0.5 mile from the trailhead, you'll notice a side canyon to your left with its own perennial water flow. Ascending this unnamed canyon for about 2 miles, then following the trail as it ascends up a draw to the left, will lead to an old ranching road. Continue up the road and through a gate at 2.5 miles from the trailhead, then on to a breccia knoll dotted with juniper that crests at 6,373 feet in elevation and offers fine views of the Salt Lake Valley to the east. If you choose to ascend to this shadeless hilltop, plan on returning the way you came up—following the road to the south will take you into Water Canyon and some private land, where your return to the trailhead is blocked by a gate and a fence.

Upon returning to Yellow Fork you can turn right and return to the trailhead, completing a 5-mile out-and-back, or turn left and continue up the canyon. If you go farther up Yellow Fork, you'll immediately pass a few picnic tables as the main trail stays near the water flow. In the spring, erythronium, or yellow fawn-lilies, bloom along the moistened canyon floor. At 1.4 miles farther up Yellow Fork, you'll come to a single picnic table—a fine place to stop for a snack or turn around. Or you can also continue even farther, eventually arriving at a dirt road that leads south and connects with an unnamed canyon. This is a popular 7-mile loop for experienced mountain bikers, but a long stretch for hikers or snowshoers.

NEARBY ACTIVITIES

Most locals don't pay much attention to the hillside mine tailings at the southwest side of the Salt Lake Valley, and many valley residents are unaware that the **Bingham Canyon Mine** (also known as the Kennecott Copper Mine) is the deepest open-pit mine in the world and the world's largest man-made excavation, at 2.5 miles wide and 0.75 mile deep. The public is welcome to come and look into the pit, learn about its history and operations, and watch the ongoing mining from a pit-side observation area. The visitor center and overlook are open to the public April 1–October 31, seven days a week, 8 a.m.–8 p.m. (you must arrive by 7 p.m. to complete the tour); call 801-204-2025 or visit **kennecott.com/visitors-center** for more information.

South: Utah County (Hikes 43–54)

Box Elder Peak

43

44 144

FS 085

Alpine Loop

FR 114

220

92 45 American Fork River

46

Cedar Hills

47 48

92

Sundance

Deer Creek Reservoir

146

Mount Timpanogos

MOUNT TIMPANOGOS WILDERNESS AREA

49

Provo River

50

S. Fork Provo River

51

89

189

52

15

Orem

265

52

53

Utah Lake

Provo

54

N

0   3   6   9 miles
0   3   6   9 kilometers

SOUTH
(UTAH COUNTY)

43 SILVER LAKE

KEY AT-A-GLANCE INFORMATION

LENGTH: 4.4 miles round-trip

ELEVATION GAIN: 1,449'

ELEVATION AT TRAILHEAD: 7,536'

CONFIGURATION: Out-and-back

DIFFICULTY: Moderate

SCENERY: Alpine lake, granite ridgeline, canyon views, woodlands

EXPOSURE: Mostly shaded for first mile, partially shaded for second

TRAFFIC: Moderate

TRAIL SURFACE: Dirt

HIKING TIME: 2.5–3.5 hours

WATER REQUIREMENTS: 1–2 liters; water from stream and lake can be purified.

SEASON: Spring, summer, fall

ACCESS: You reach the hike, which lies within the Lone Peak Wilderness Area, through American Fork Canyon, a fee-access area (see page 4). No parking fees.

MAPS: USGS Dromedary Peak, Trails Illustrated Uinta National Forest (701)

FACILITIES: Restrooms at trailhead

DOGS: On leash

SPECIAL COMMENTS: No mechanized vehicles, bikes, or horses are permitted on the trail.

GPS TRAILHEAD COORDINATES

N40° 30.420´ W111° 39.380´

IN BRIEF

Breathtaking alpine scenery, abundant wildlife, and a well-designed new trail to a blue lake nestled in a glacial bowl make Silver Lake one of the most perfect hikes in Utah County. It's a great day hike, but you'll want to stay longer.

DESCRIPTION

What begins as a pleasant and shaded uphill stroll concludes with one of the most dramatic wilderness settings in Utah. You'll think you've been transported to Yosemite in the Sierra Nevada. It has all the iconic elements of that far-more-famous national park: towering gray-granite walls, blue glacial lakes, spruce and fir trees, cascading waterfalls, glistening streams, and moose—lots of moose.

The 3 miles of dirt road leading to the trailhead and its location within the Lone Peak Wilderness Area discourage many less-serious hikers from visiting Silver Lake. As a result, the hike is not as crowded as one might expect for a jewel of this magnitude. The dirt road from Granite Flat to the trailhead at Silver

----

Directions

From Salt Lake City, take I-15 south to Highland/Alpine (Exit 284). At the bottom of the off-ramp, turn left on UT 92 and continue east 12.4 miles to the junction of UT 92 and UT 144 (FR 085). Turn left onto UT 144 toward Tibble Fork. Continue 2.5 miles on UT 144, to the east end of Tibble Fork Reservoir. Turn left onto the paved road going up to Granite Flat Campground. After 0.7 mile, turn right onto Forest Service Road 008 toward Silver Lake Flat, immediately before entering the Granite Flat Campground. Continue 3.2 miles on this dirt road to Silver Lake Flat, where you'll find trailhead parking on your left, at the north end of the lake.

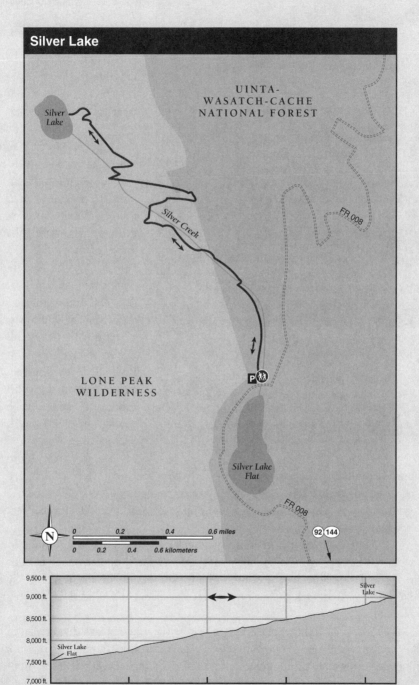

Silver Lake

Silver Lake

UINTA-
WASATCH-CACHE
NATIONAL FOREST

FR 008

Silver Creek

LONE PEAK
WILDERNESS

P

Silver Lake
Flat

FR 008

92 144

N

| 0 | 0.2 | 0.4 | 0.6 miles |

| 0 | 0.2 | 0.4 | 0.6 kilometers |

Silver
Lake

Silver Lake
Flat

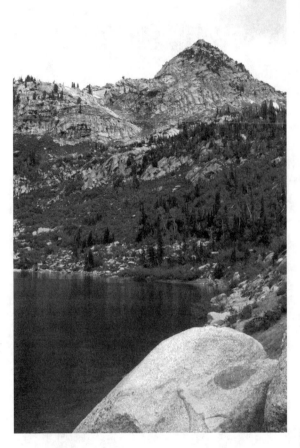

Silver Lake, with White Baldy in the background

Lake Flat is rugged but passable for most passenger vehicles—just watch out for large, protruding rocks.

From the trailhead parking area on the north side of Silver Lake Flat reservoir, take the well-marked trail to the right of the restrooms. The trail ascends through a beautiful, shaded grove of aspen dotted with Douglas-fir. Large granite boulders, many the size of cars, also appear throughout the Silver Creek drainage.

Birds fill the woodland in the spring and summer. Red-tailed hawks and golden eagles nest in the conifers; American robins and black-headed grosbeaks share the deciduous groves.

At 0.4 mile from the trailhead, you'll pass a clearing on the right where beavers have leveled an acre or so of aspen for their dams. At 0.5 mile, you enter the Lone Peak Wilderness Area, marked by a sign. Throughout this lower drainage, you can often see deer feeding on the lush undergrowth.

At 1.1 miles the trail rises above the creek and moves up the dry slope to the east. As you emerge from the shade of the aspens, you'll find striking views of the canyons and ridgeline to the south. Along this section of the trail, watch for chokecherry bushes with their white flowers in spring and reddish-purple berries in summer.

When you reach the upper drainage, below the granite bowl that cradles Silver Lake, you may well spot both mountain goats and moose. Remember that a large bull moose can weigh 1,200 pounds and stand more than 7 feet tall at the shoulder. Because these animals can be temperamental and aggressive—and will charge at high speeds if provoked—you should avoid approaching them and keep a safe distance. Don't come between a moose cow and her calf, or between a moose and the water.

Just below Silver Lake, you'll pass a cascading waterfall along Silver Creek to the left as it drains from the lake. Subalpine fir makes its appearance at this higher elevation. Within 5 minutes you crest the large granite boulders that form the rim of the lake, and you've instantly arrived at the shore. Depending on the amount of snowfall and the spring temperatures, Silver Lake may well be frozen into May, and occasionally into June.

By quickly scanning the shore, you'll often spot moose grazing on the aquatic plant life in the lake. Also, keep your eyes peeled for mountain goats on the rocky slopes above the lake. The Yosemite-quality granite cathedral towering over the northeast side of the lake is White Baldy. At 11,321 feet, it is one of the higher but least-visited peaks on the ridge. A good scramble that is typically approached from Red Pine Lake in Little Cottonwood Canyon, the White Baldy hike can also be approached from Silver Lake.

Once you've hiked the 2.2 miles from the trailhead to the shores of Silver Lake, circle the lake through the maze of granite boulders at its rim. You can also ascend another 0.7 mile and 900 vertical feet to the northeast and discover the smaller Silver Glance Lake with an even rockier, more rugged setting. But most visitors are content to find a natural granite countertop on which to enjoy a snack and take in the mesmerizing beauty of this alpine treasure.

NEARBY ACTIVITIES

American Fork Canyon is a year-round scenic wonder and recreational playground that's popular with all types and all ages of outdoor enthusiasts. You'll find a wide range of camping options, with wilderness and improved campgrounds, as well as many picnic and day-use facilities. Hiking, rock climbing, fishing, ATV riding, snowmobiling, cross-country skiing, horseback riding, and mountain biking are all popular pursuits here.

44 BOX ELDER PEAK

IN BRIEF

One of the lesser-known big peaks of the Wasatch, Box Elder Peak offers exceptional mountain-wilderness scenery and wildlife-viewing. Most fit hikers can achieve the adventurous off-trail scramble to the summit.

DESCRIPTION

Tucked amid slightly larger and more frequently climbed peaks, including Lone Peak, Pfeiffer-horn, and Mount Timpanogos, Box Elder Peak is easily overlooked—even with its 11,101-foot triangular summit. Although marked trails ring the peak, no maintained trail leads to the summit. As a result, Box Elder gives hikers the opportunity to enjoy a stunning alpine wilderness setting at the lower elevations and then experience the challenge of a summit quest involving some scrambling and route-finding on rarely used routes.

You can access the trails around Box Elder Peak from Alpine to the west or from American Fork Canyon to the east. Most people who set out to climb the peak use the Deer Creek–Dry Creek Trail (#043) and either start at an elevation of 5,600 feet in Alpine or at

---

Directions _____

From Salt Lake City, take I-15 south to High-land/Alpine (Exit 284). At the bottom of the off-ramp, turn left and take UT 92 east 12.4 miles to the junction of UT 92 and UT 144 (FR 085). Turn left onto UT 144 toward Tibble Fork. Continue 2.5 miles on UT 144, to the east end of Tibble Fork Reservoir. Turn left onto the paved road going up to Granite Flat and enter the campground at 0.7 mile. You'll find trailhead parking to the right of the road, at the Sandwagon Group Site. The trailhead is at the north end of the parking lot.

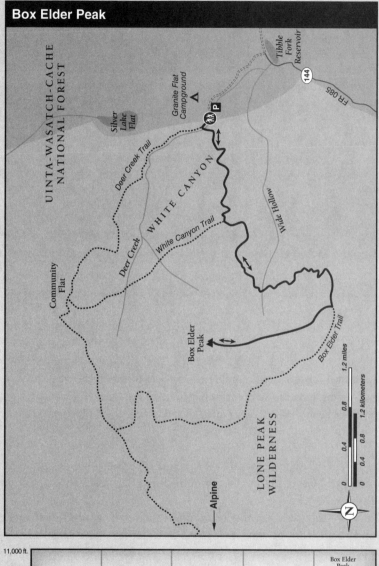

Box Elder Peak

UINTA-WASATCH-CACHE NATIONAL FOREST

Tibble Fork Reservoir

144

FR 085

Silver Lake Flat

Granite Flat Campground

P

Deer Creek Trail

WHITE CANYON

Deer Creek

White Canyon Trail

Wide Hollow

Community Flat

Box Elder Peak

Box Elder Trail

LONE PEAK WILDERNESS

Alpine

1.2 miles

0.8

0.4

0

1.2 kilometers

0.8

0.4

0

N

11,000 ft.

10,000 ft.

9,000 ft.

8,000 ft.

7,000 ft.

6,000 ft.

Box Elder Peak

Granite Flat

1 mi.   2 mi.   3 mi.   4 mi.   4.9 mi.

Photo: Gina Duncan

Mountain goat in American Fork Canyon

the 6,778-foot level at Granite Flat. They then approach the peak from the north side. The advantage of taking the Box Elder Trail along the southern flanks of the peak is that it offers a more favorable ridge route to the summit and makes getting lost or dropping into the wrong drainage less likely on the descent. Additionally, the Box Elder Peak Trail offers greater solitude, better wildlife-viewing, and some less frequently visited mountain scenery along the way.

Within 100 yards of the trailhead, you'll pass a sign marking your entrance into the Lone Peak Wilderness Area. Moments later you come to a junction of the Deer Creek–Dry Creek Trail (#043) and the Box Elder Trail (#044). Take the Box Elder Trail to the left.

The path rises steeply through successively higher meadows linked by stands of aspen and conifer, but no box-elder trees. By entering these meadows slowly and quietly, visually scanning the rim, you'll have a good chance of spotting deer and occasionally moose. At 1.8 miles, you'll come to a natural spring trickling down the side of a rock to the right of the trail. At 2.3 miles, you'll see the remains of an old cabin on the left side of the trail. This cabin must have been "property with a view," as it's perched near a ledge overlooking Wide Hollow, a deep, glacial side canyon.

Shortly after passing the cabin, you'll come to a sign marking the White Canyon Trail (#188), which heads north and connects with the Deer Creek–Dry Creek Trail. Stay on the Box Elder Peak Trail to the left as it dips into Wide Hollow and crosses the seasonal runoff. As the trail crosses Wide Hollow and rises above the 8,700-foot level, you leave the mostly shaded woodland for partially shaded alpine meadows and ridges. Snowpack often remains into midsummer in the bowls and on the north-facing slopes at these higher elevations. You're in wilderness, and along the trail you're just as likely to see bear tracks as boot tracks. It's important to trust the trail, since the route is unintuitive and the summit doesn't come into sight until you cross the upper ridge.

When you arrive at the saddle, views of the Utah Valley open to the west. The trail continues to the northwest along a level contour near 9,700 feet. Here you'll see the summit, and you must determine the best place to depart the trail and head for it. One good choice appears after crossing a steep shale slope. A faint ridgeline leads up to the northwest, and while the ascent is steep, it provides better footing than some of the scree slopes.

On the way to the summit, and often once you're there, you can see a herd of mountain goats that find safety from predators in this high, rocky terrain. From the summit, you have good views of Utah Valley but excellent ones of Mount Timpanogos to the south and Lone Peak and Pfeifferhorn ridge to the north.

If the summit isn't your ultimate destination, you can also continue circling Box Elder Peak clockwise, eventually connecting with the Deer Creek–Dry Creek Trail and returning to the Granite Flat trailhead. After all, Box Elder Peak isn't just about the summit—it's a wilderness experience and an adventure in mountain solitude.

Note: Mechanized vehicles and bikes are prohibited in the Lone Peak Wilderness Area.

NEARBY ACTIVITIES

The city of Alpine, settled in 1850 by Mormon pioneers under the name of Mountainville, lies at the base of Box Elder Peak. Today, it's a growing residential community proud of its rural roots. The **Petersen Arboretum,** in Petersen Park at Ridge Drive and 100 East, features hundreds of trees of both native and non-native species.

45 TIMPANOGOS CAVE NATIONAL MONUMENT

KEY AT-A-GLANCE INFORMATION

LENGTH: 3 miles round-trip

ELEVATION GAIN: 1,092'

ELEVATION AT TRAILHEAD: 5,638'

CONFIGURATION: Out-and-back

DIFFICULTY: Moderate

SCENERY: Riparian canyon with rock cliffs and subalpine slopes leading to cave

EXPOSURE: Mostly shaded to 8,000', partially shaded to 9,000', fully exposed above 9,000'

TRAFFIC: Busy

TRAIL SURFACE: Paved

HIKING TIME: 1–2.5 hours on trail + 1 additional hour for cave tour

WATER REQUIREMENTS: 1 liter; no water on trail

SEASON: Early May–early October

ACCESS: The hike lies within Timpanogos Cave National Monument in American Fork Canyon, a fee-access area (see page 4). There is no charge to hike the cave trail. Tickets for cave tours are sold at the visitor center (see page 4). The trail and caves are closed early October–early May.

MAPS: USGS Timpanogos Cave, Trails Illustrated Uinta National Forest (701)

FACILITIES: Restrooms, phones, water, snack stand, gift shop, and visitor center at trailhead; vault toilet along trail near cave entrance

DOGS: Prohibited on trail; kennel facilities available for hikers with dogs

GPS TRAILHEAD COORDINATES

N40° 26.607´ W111° 42.298´

IN BRIEF

This spectacular trail is carved into and through rocky cliffs that rise high above American Fork Canyon. The trail ascends 1,000 feet of canyon wall to arrive at the entrance of Timpanogos Cave. The trail alone is worth the admission price to the cave. A perfect summer outing and must-see destination.

DESCRIPTION

Even if this weren't a national monument with a fascinating cave system awaiting at the end of the short paved trail, this would still be an exceptional hike. It takes you from the American Fork River on the canyon floor, up sheer rock cliffs exposing millions of years of geology, and through a subalpine forest of fir and pine, with breathtaking canyon views all along the way.

In 1887, long before anyone thought of building a trail up the canyon cliffs, settler Martin Hansen was cutting timber high on the slopes of American Fork Canyon. He noticed mountain-lion tracks leading up the hillside and followed them to a high ledge, where he found an opening in the limestone cliff to a small cave. This cave was the first of three linked caverns that contain about 2 miles of underground passages filled with colorful limestone deposits and clear-water pools.

- -

Directions ⟶

From Salt Lake City, take I-15 south to Highland/Alpine (Exit 284). At the end of the offramp, turn left and continue east 10 miles on UT 92 to the Timpanogos Cave National Monument parking area and visitor center, on the right. The trailhead is on the east side of the visitor center.

Timpanogos Cave National Monument

Swinging Bridge Creek

UINTA-WASATCH-CACHE
NATIONAL FOREST

Visitor
Center

92

American Fork River

Alpine Scenic Highway

92

TIMPANOGOS CAVE
NATIONAL
MONUMENT

cave exit

cave
entrance

N

| 0 | 0.1 | 0.2 | 0.3 miles |

| 0 | 0.1 | 0.2 | 0.3 kilometers |

7,500 ft.						
7,000 ft.					Cave Entrance	Cave Exit
6,500 ft.						
6,000 ft.						
5,500 ft.	Visitor Center					
5,000 ft.	0.25 mi.	0.5 mi.	0.75 mi.	1 mi.	1.25 mi.	1.5 mi.

The trail includes several well-developed switchbacks.

Miners and early visitors stripped the center cave of many of its slow-growing formations. At one point, two railroad freight cars filled with flowstone were shipped to the east. But the discovery of two adjoining caves and the protection granted by the National Park Service in 1934 ensure that these fragile underground wonders will be available for us and future generations to enjoy.

During its five-month operating season, Timpanogos Cave National Monument hosts around 70,000 visitors from all over the world. Most of those guests hike the trail because it's the only way to get to the cave. Thousands of additional visitors come just to hike the trail as part of a regular exercise program. The hike to the cave entrance is a good test of your conditioning and readiness for other, more strenuous hikes. If the point of your visit is to see the cave, make sure you allow yourself time to enjoy the trail and read the interpretive signs along the way.

The fact that the trail is paved doesn't detract one bit from the pristine beauty of the canyon wall. In fact, you'll appreciate the sure-footed surface, especially as you pass numerous unprotected drop-offs where a simple misstep could prove fatal. The caves are closed when weather makes hiking to them difficult or dangerous. No strollers or wheelchairs are allowed on the trail. Some sections of the trail are particularly susceptible to rockfall and are marked by a red stripe. No stopping or standing is allowed in these areas.

A hike to the caves is a field course in Wasatch geology, with an open display of sedimentary and metamorphic layers, uplifted layers, and an active fault. Starting at the trailhead, you'll pass through an initial layer of quartzite, followed by distinctive layers of shale, limestone, dolomite, and finally two layers of beautiful black limestone embedded with fossils of sea creatures and other remains of plant and animal life.

A steep cliffside trail leads to the cave.

The canyon cliffs support an amazing range of conifers, many of which cling to the rocky ledges with twisted and gnarled exposed roots. Douglas-fir, white fir, and limber pine line the trail; scrub oak and bigtooth maple fill in the gaps.

Wildlife sightings on the trail are uncommon, but don't be surprised by chipmunks and squirrels along the way, or even an occasional rattlesnake on the rocky ledges. Looking across the canyon, you can often see red-tailed hawks and golden eagles soaring above. Bird-watchers may find their best opportunities on the Swinging Bridge Nature Trail across the road from the visitor center. The riverside vegetation is home to brightly colored western tanagers, Steller's jays, canyon wrens, and American dippers.

Allow 1.5–2 hours on the trail, plus an additional hour for the ranger-guided cave tour. Even when canyon temperatures hover in the 90s, the temperature in the cave remains a constant 45°F. Since you'll be in the cave for about an hour, make sure you come prepared with warm clothing for the tour. After completing the tour, you'll exit at the east end of the cave and follow a short loop back to the main trail for your descent.

NEARBY ACTIVITIES

A visit to **Timpanogos Cave National Monument** is typically centered around a cave tour. In summer, all tours usually sell out by early afternoon. Buy tickets in advance at the visitor center, or arrive early in the day to avoid long delays or disappointment. While waiting for your tour to depart, you can watch the introductory video at the visitor center, enjoy the picnic areas across the street, or explore the 0.25-mile nature trail. For reservations and information, call 801-756-5238 or visit **nps.gov/tica**.

46 MOUNT TIMPANOGOS
(via the Timpooneke Trail)

KEY AT-A-GLANCE INFORMATION

LENGTH: 13 miles round-trip to saddle and back, 14.8 miles round-trip to summit and back

ELEVATION GAIN: 4,389' to summit

ELEVATION AT TRAILHEAD: 7,360'

CONFIGURATION: Out-and-back

DIFFICULTY: Hard

SCENERY: Mountain scenery, glacial basins, flowered meadows, lakes, and valley views

EXPOSURE: Mostly shaded below 8,000', partially shaded to 9,500', fully exposed above 9,500'

TRAFFIC: Busy

TRAIL SURFACE: Dirt and rock to saddle, exclusively rock from saddle to summit

HIKING TIME: 6–11 hours

WATER REQUIREMENTS: 2–3 liters; water from lake, streams, springs, and snowmelt can be purified.

SEASON: Late spring, summer, early fall

ACCESS: The trail is accessed from American Fork Canyon, a fee-access area (see page 4). No parking fees.

MAPS: USGS Timpanogos Cave, Trails Illustrated Uinta National Forest (701)

FACILITIES: Restrooms and water at trailhead; toilet near trail at Timpanogos Basin

DOGS: Permitted

GPS TRAILHEAD COORDINATES

N40° 25.878´ W111° 38.328´

IN BRIEF

The Timpanogos massif dominates the skyline of Utah County. At 11,749 feet, this majestic peak is the second highest in the Wasatch (just below Mount Nebo to the south, at 11,928 feet). But looking at the steep, barren, western slope of Mount Timpanogos, it's hard to imagine the spectacular beauty to be found on the expansive, wooded eastern slopes, where trails lead past glistening lakes, flowered meadows, cascading waterfalls, and on to the summit.

DESCRIPTION

Mount Timpanogos, or "Timp" for short, is the most popular mountain-hiking destination in Utah. On any given summer Saturday, between 700 and 1,000 hikers depart from the two trailheads leading to the summit. Many have a summit destination in mind, and typically about 200–300 of those hikers make it to the top of the 11,749-foot peak. Some hikers make their ultimate destination one of the many waterfalls, meadows, or lakes, while others go as far as the saddle, less than a mile from the summit, and consider the view from the saddle as a worthy reward for their effort.

A frequent topic of discussion among Timp hikers is, "Which is the best trail to the summit: Aspen Grove or Timpooneke?" Truth is, the routes are equally popular, with about as many starting on one as the other. Each

Directions

From Salt Lake City, go south on I-15 to Highland/Alpine (Exit 284). At the bottom of the off-ramp, turn left on UT 92 and proceed 18 miles to the Timpooneke Campground. Turn right into the campground and continue 0.3 mile to the trailhead parking lot, on the left.

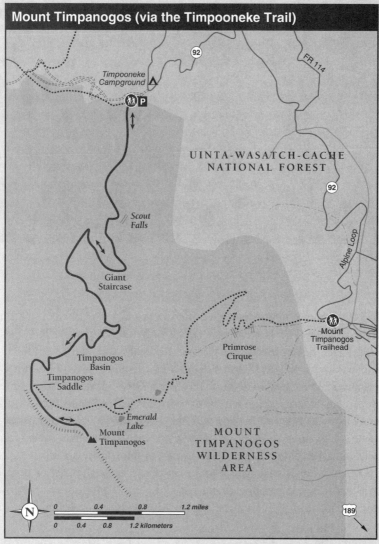

Mount Timpanogos (via the Timpooneke Trail)

Timpooneke
Campground

92

FR 114

UINTA-WASATCH-CACHE
NATIONAL FOREST

92

Alpine Loop

Scout
Falls

Giant
Staircase

Primrose
Cirque

Mount
Timpanogos
Trailhead

Timpanogos
Basin

Timpanogos
Saddle

Emerald
Lake

Mount
Timpanogos

MOUNT
TIMPANOGOS
WILDERNESS
AREA

N

| 0 | 0.4 | 0.8 | 1.2 miles |
| 0 | 0.4 | 0.8 | 1.2 kilometers |

189

16,000 ft.

14,000 ft.

12,000 ft.

10,000 ft.

8,000 ft.

6,000 ft.

Summit

Saddle

Timpanogos
Basin

Great
Staircase

Timpooneke
Trailhead

2 mi.   4 mi.   6 mi.   7.4 mi.

Photo: Rob Witt

Hikers descend the Timpooneke Trail.

route arrives at the saddle from a different direction, but they share the final 0.9 mile to the summit. The Timpooneke Trail is only 0.6 mile longer than the Aspen Grove Trail (see next profile), but Timpooneke has the gentler grade, since its starting elevation is 471 feet higher than that of Aspen Grove. The Timpooneke Trail ascends 593 feet per mile, while the Aspen Grove Trail ascends 714 feet per mile. Both offer comparable scenery—the Aspen Grove Trail climbs the gaping Primrose Cirque to Emerald Lake, while the Timpooneke Trail ascends the Giant Staircase to Timpanogos Basin. Admittedly, Aspen Grove has more accessible waterfalls and lakes along the trail, which add to the enjoyment of the hike.

For most hikers it's a toss-up, and many experience the best of both routes by leaving a car at each trailhead and hiking up the Timpooneke and down the Aspen Grove. Either way, it's a great hike and the quintessential climb to a Wasatch mountain summit.

Climbing Timp can make for a long day, so an early start—even before dawn— can work to your advantage. This is especially important if you're not acclimatized to the high elevations and you're forced to move a little more slowly. In summer, starting early enables you to gain most of your elevation in the shade, before the sun comes over the mountain and casts its direct rays. Also, on weekends and holidays the Timpooneke trailhead parking lot can fill by 7 a.m., and you may be forced to park a mile or more away at an additional cost. As you might imagine, the Timpooneke Trail can be a bustling thoroughfare on weekends, so if you want a bit of mountain solitude, plan a midweek hike.

From the trailhead parking area, sign the register and begin your climb on Trail #053 through woods of Douglas-fir. The trail ascends a tiered drainage along a series of five benches known as the Giant Staircase. The Timpanogos massif is composed almost entirely of gray Oquirrh limestone, with alternating layers of limestone, sandstone, and shale exposed in the upper reaches of the mountain.

Each of the benches along the Giant Staircase becomes more open and is accompanied by a meadow of wildflowers. Finally at the upper basin, known as the Timpanogos Basin, hikers are exposed to a riot of wildflowers, with alpine aster, white columbine, Parry's primrose, and larkspur providing a colorful foreground to views of the summit directly to the south. At this point, the elevation is 10,200 feet and the remaining hike to the summit is above tree line along rocky slopes.

On the north side of the basin, you'll come to a trail marker pointing to a backcountry toilet to the right, while the main trail continues straight ahead. Following the spur to the toilet also leads you to the wreckage of a B-25 airplane that crashed in the basin in 1955. The two engines and some sections of the fuselage remain. Continuing up a switchback on this slope, you'll come to a small cascade descending from snowmelt on an upper bowl. This is your last access to water before heading on to the summit.

As you ascend the rocky slope to the saddle, notice a steep trail descending on the left and to the south. This trail leads across a boulder field, often covered with snow, to Emerald Lake and the Aspen Grove Trail. Hikers coming up the Aspen Grove Trail to the summit typically use this steep trail to reach the saddle. A few minutes after passing this junction, you'll arrive at the saddle.

The Timpanogos saddle, at an elevation of 11,050 feet, offers excellent views of Utah Valley to the west. It's a popular gathering place and comfortable rest stop—so comfortable that many hikers make it their final destination without going to the summit. Continuing on to the summit requires another 0.9 mile of steady and sometimes steep ascents along a well-crafted rocky trail. A steady pace should take you from the saddle to the summit in 35 minutes, but most hikers frequently stop to catch their breath, and the trip takes between 45 minutes and 1 hour to gain 700 vertical feet to the metal summit hut.

You can expect your return trip to be faster than your ascent, but be particularly careful descending the loose scree below the summit. Once below the saddle you'll find the trail provides a surefooted gradual descent, but with afternoon sun beaming down on exposed slopes, you'll want plenty of sunscreen and water.

NEARBY ACTIVITIES

The 20-mile **Alpine Loop Scenic Backway** (UT 92) passes through canyons and forests of aspen and Douglas-fir. It goes up American Fork Canyon and continues through Uinta-Wasatch-Cache National Forest to Provo Canyon. Open late May–late October, the road affords wonderful views of fall colors. When snow closes part of the road in winter, it becomes a favorite snowmobiling and cross-country-skiing trail. The narrow, winding road is not recommended for vehicles more than 30 feet long.

47 EMERALD LAKE AND MOUNT TIMPANOGOS (via Aspen Grove Trail)

KEY AT-A-GLANCE INFORMATION

LENGTH: 9.6 miles round-trip to Emerald Lake and back, 13.6 miles round-trip to Mt. Timpanogos summit and back

ELEVATION GAIN: 3,491' to Emerald Lake, 4,860' to Mt. Timpanogos summit

ELEVATION AT TRAILHEAD: 6,889'

CONFIGURATION: Out-and-back

DIFFICULTY: Hard

SCENERY: Mountain scenery, glacial basins, flowered meadows, lakes, valley views

EXPOSURE: Partially shaded to 9,500', fully exposed above 9,500'

TRAFFIC: Busy

TRAIL SURFACE: Asphalt for first mile, dirt and rock to Emerald Lake, mostly rock to summit

HIKING TIME: 4.5–7 hours to Emerald Lake, 7–11 hours to summit

WATER REQUIREMENTS: 2–3 liters; water in streams, springs, lakes, and snowfields along trail can be purified.

SEASON: Summer–early fall

ACCESS: The trail is accessed from the Aspen Grove trailhead on the Alpine Loop Scenic Backway, a fee-access area (see page 4).

MAPS: USGS Timpanogos Cave, Trails Illustrated Uinta National Forest (701)

FACILITIES: Restrooms and water at trailhead

DOGS: On leash

GPS TRAILHEAD COORDINATES

N40° 24.263´ W111° 36.323´

IN BRIEF

The Mount Timpanogos Wilderness Area is full of superlatives. Whether you're hiking to a waterfall in Primrose Cirque, an alpine meadow, Emerald Lake, the Timpanogos snowfield, or on to the summit, you'll find plenty to grab your attention and make you want to go higher and farther.

DESCRIPTION

The Aspen Grove Trail, like its sister, the Timpooneke Trail (see previous profile), leads up an immense drainage to a glacial bowl, then on to the saddle and summit of Mount Timpanogos. While both are great trails and offer a challenging, spectacular, and often-overcrowded wilderness experience, the Aspen Grove Trail provides more access to water (in the form of waterfalls, streams, lakes, and snowfields) than the Timpooneke Trail. The Aspen Grove Trail also has more vertical elevation gain and is slightly shorter and steeper than the Timpooneke Trail. Finally, it offers a better chance of seeing the herd of mountain goats that call "Timp" home.

Directions ————————————————→

From Salt Lake City, go south on I-15 to Orem 800 North (Exit 272). At the bottom of the off-ramp, turn left and proceed east 3.7 miles on 800 North (UT 52) toward the mouth of Provo Canyon. Take the left ramp onto East Provo Canyon Road (US 189). Continue up the canyon for 7 miles to UT 92, the first left after the tunnel. Continue up UT 92, passing Sundance and the Aspen Grove Family Camp on the left. Pass the Forest Service fee booth at 4.6 miles and enter the trailhead parking lot, immediately on the left.

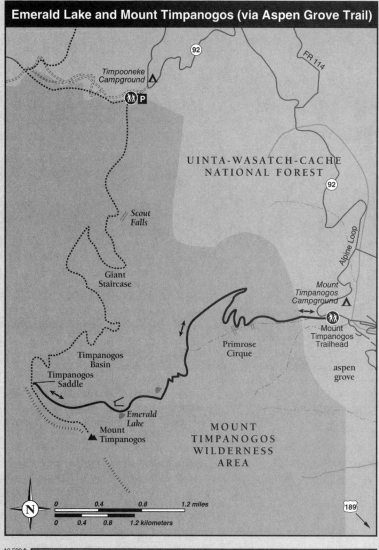

Emerald Lake and Mount Timpanogos (via Aspen Grove Trail)

92

FR 114

Timpooneke Campground △

UINTA-WASATCH-CACHE NATIONAL FOREST

92

Scout Falls

Alpine Loop

Giant Staircase

Mount Timpanogos Campground △

Mount Timpanogos Trailhead

Timpanogos Basin

Primrose Cirque

aspen grove

Timpanogos Saddle

Emerald Lake

Mount ▲ Timpanogos

MOUNT TIMPANOGOS WILDERNESS AREA

N

| 0 | 0.4 | 0.8 | 1.2 miles |
| 0 | 0.4 | 0.8 | 1.2 kilometers |

189

13,500 ft.								Summit
12,000 ft.				↔	Emerald Lake			
10,500 ft.								
9,000 ft.								
7,500 ft.	Primrose Cirque							
6,000 ft.			2 mi.		4 mi.		6 mi.	6.8 mi.

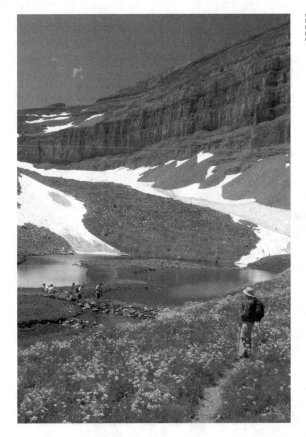

Emerald Lake

The name *Timpanogos* (timp-ah-NO-gus) comes from the Paiute name for the Provo River, meaning "rock and running water." It has nothing to do with a silly legend contrived in the early 20th century, which holds that the image of a lovesick Indian maiden who threw herself off the peak can still be seen in the mountain skyline.

The trail departs from the north side of the large Theater in the Pines parking area and passes a small guard station, where you should sign in during the peak summer season. The trail gradually ascends the lower drainage through woods of quaking aspen and Douglas-fir. To the left is a steep avalanche slope where thousands of trees have been leveled and several lives have been lost in recent avalanches.

After entering the Mount Timpanogos Wilderness Area, the trail is paved in asphalt for the next mile. The trail arrives at a waterfall on the left, then makes a sharp turn to the right and into some switchbacks before arriving at a second waterfall. Here the asphalt ends and the trail begins a giant, gradually ascending sweep to the east along the partially shaded south-facing slope of Primrose Cirque. At about 8,000 feet in elevation, the trail turns sharply back to the west and continues its climb of the expansive cirque. Along the way, the trail traverses rocky slopes and passes by several waterfalls and small runoffs.

This section of trail can be particularly treacherous in the spring and early summer, as melting snowfields form ice bridges across the flowing water. Falling through these snowfields to the rocks and rushing water below has resulted in injuries and deaths for unprepared hikers. Use extreme caution when crossing some of the steep snowfields in this section of the trail.

After winding your way up the limestone terraces at the top of Primrose Cirque, you'll pass through a grove of Engelmann spruce (a popular camping area) at an elevation of about 9,500 feet, then move on to a high meadow laced with streams and small lakes. After several stream crossings, the trail ascends to the crest of a moraine slope and the Timpanogos Shelter comes into view, followed by views of Emerald Lake.

Emerald Lake is a wonderful destination if you've made a late start or want a shorter, less demanding outing. The shelter provides the only shade in the area, and a recently constructed toilet lies along a path to the northeast of the shelter.

The Timpanogos Shelter, just 100 yards to the north of Emerald Lake, was built in 1959 by the U.S. Forest Service. From 1959 to 1970 it was used as part of the Timp Hike, a community event that drew thousands to the mountain each year on a single late-July weekend. The hike was discontinued in 1970 in an effort to preserve the delicate mountain environment.

Rising to the west of Emerald Lake toward the ridgeline is the Timpanogos Glacier. Whether it's an actual glacier or not has been the subject of some debate: Trip reports from the early 20th century note the existence of crevasses, indicative of a true glacier. The Dust Bowl drought of the 1930s diminished the glacier considerably, and throughout most of the 20th century it waxed and waned with variations in annual snowfall and temperatures. But in 1994, the snowfield melted sufficiently to reveal some glacial ice below the talus. Studies were inconclusive, so the debate rages on regarding whether it's a glacier, a permanent snowfield, or just a patch of snow. The snowfield can be used for both a summit ascent in the spring (typically requiring ice ax and crampons) and for a glissade descent in the summer. Sliding down the snowfield is a popular, fast, and increasingly dangerous descent route. Examine conditions carefully, and use caution.

The route from the shelter to the saddle crosses the meadow north of Emerald Lake to a boulder field often covered with large patches of snow. The area around Emerald Lake is your best opportunity to spot mountain goats that often graze in the meadow and find an easy retreat to the high rocky ledges of Mount Timpanogos. Mountain goats found in Utah are a nonnative species introduced in 1967 from a herd in Washington's Olympic National Park. In addition to Mount Timpanogos, they have been successfully transplanted to the Cottonwood Canyons, the Uintas, and the Tushar Mountains in southern Utah. The current population statewide is more than 1,000, with about 200 inhabiting the Timpanogos massif.

The most grueling section of trail rises from the boulder field above the Timpanogos Basin and steeply ascends to the north before joining the Timpooneke Trail and continuing to the saddle. From the saddle, it's a demanding, rocky 0.9-mile climb to the metal shelter at the 11,749-foot summit. Here you'll have commanding views of Utah Valley to the west and Heber Valley to the east.

Mount Timpanogos is arguably the best mountain hike in Utah, and certainly a classic that every local hiker should experience. As with most mountains, summit success favors those who get an early start. Once you've returned to Emerald Lake from the summit, the afternoon descent along the sunny slopes of Primrose Cirque can be long and hot, so bring plenty of water and sunscreen.

48 STEWART FALLS

KEY AT-A-GLANCE INFORMATION

LENGTH: 3.6 miles round-trip

ELEVATION GAIN: 310'

ELEVATION AT TRAILHEAD: 6,889'

CONFIGURATION: Out-and-back

DIFFICULTY: Easy

SCENERY: Mountain views and waterfall

EXPOSURE: Mostly shaded for first mile, partially shaded for second

TRAFFIC: Busy

TRAIL SURFACE: Dirt

HIKING TIME: 1.5–2.5 hours

WATER REQUIREMENTS: 1 liter; water in the stream below the falls can be purified.

SEASON: Spring, summer, fall

ACCESS: The Aspen Grove trailhead parking area lies within the Alpine Loop Scenic Backway fee-access area (see page 4), while the trail itself is almost entirely on Sundance Resort property. Stewart Falls lies within the Mount Timpanogos Wilderness Area.

MAPS: USGS Aspen Grove, Trails Illustrated Uinta National Forest (701)

FACILITIES: Restrooms and drinking water at trailhead parking area

DOGS: On leash

SPECIAL COMMENTS: Sections of this hike are avalanche-prone and should not be attempted in winter.

GPS TRAILHEAD COORDINATES

N40° 24.263´ W111° 36.323´

IN BRIEF

A tiered wedding cake of cascading water set against a mountain backdrop of aspen and fir, Stewart Falls may be the most picturesque waterfall in Utah. The gentle trail is well suited for families, making this an ideal three-season day hike.

DESCRIPTION

For the thousands of Utah Valley residents living below the western slopes of the Timpanogos massif, it's easy to forget how incredibly beautiful the "back side of Timp" is. They should be required to pay a visit at least twice a year—spring, summer, fall, winter; it doesn't matter—to walk through the aspens, breathe the mountain air, and sit by a mountain stream at the base of a thundering waterfall.

Mount Timpanogos boasts some exquisite waterfalls on all sides, and the falls along both Aspen Grove Trail and the Timpooneke Trail should be on every hiker's must-see list. But Stewart Falls, sometimes referred to as Stewarts Cascades, is the most beautiful and accessible of them all. In less than 2 miles from the trailhead, walking along a well-groomed

----

Directions

From Salt Lake City, go south on I-15 to Orem 800 North (Exit 272). At the bottom of the off-ramp, turn left and proceed east 3.7 miles on 800 North (UT 52) toward the mouth of Provo Canyon. Take the left ramp onto East Provo Canyon Road (US 189). Continue 7 miles up the canyon to UT 92, the first left after the tunnel. Continue up UT 92, passing Sundance and the Aspen Grove Family Camp on the left. Pass the U.S. Forest Service fee booth at 4.6 miles and enter the trailhead parking lot, immediately on the left.

Stewart Falls

Alpine Loop

92

Mount Timpanogos
Campground

Emerald
Lake

P

aspen
grove

92

UINTA-WASATCH-CACHE
NATIONAL FOREST

MOUNT
TIMPANOGOS
WILDERNESS
AREA

N

| 0 | 0.1 | 0.2 | 0.3 miles |

| 0 | 0.1 | 0.2 | 0.3 kilometers |

89

7,300 ft.
7,200 ft.
7,100 ft.
7,000 ft.
6,900 ft.
6,800 ft.

Aspen Grove
Trailhead

Stewart
Falls

0.5 mi.   1 mi.   1.5 mi.   1.8 mi.

Stewart Falls

Photo: Ahmad Asgharzadeh/iStockPhoto.com

wooded slope, you find yourself face-to-face with tiers of cascading spring water.

From the large trailhead parking area, take the trail to the right of the restroom that leads up Primrose Cirque. Follow the sign marked STEWART FALLS, TRAIL 56. As you look at the slope in front of you to the left, you can see the damage done by recent avalanches that resulted in the loss of several lives. At 0.1 mile, the trail turns sharply to the left and ascends the hillside through a forest of Douglas-fir and aspen. At 1.2 miles, the path passes through the middle of an avalanche slope where hundreds of aspens have been leveled.

Along the way you'll find a rich variety of birds in the trees and underbrush. Yellow-bellied sapsuckers, mountain bluebirds, yellow warblers, and western tanagers are just a few of the colorful varieties you may see. Squirrels make their home in the underbrush of scrub oak, bigtooth maple, and Oregon grape.

The trail reaches a peak elevation of 7,200 feet before beginning its descent toward the falls. Soon the roar of the falls can be heard even before they come into view. At 1.5 miles from the trailhead, as you come around a bend, your first view of Stewart Falls awaits. Another cascade plunges down the slope to the right.

At 1.7 miles from the trailhead, you'll come to a shale outcrop that serves as a great falls overlook. From there, take the marked trail that descends to the left. A few short switchbacks lead you to the stream level at the base of the falls. Plenty of great vantage points below the falls offer places to play in the water or enjoy a snack. However, the barren slope to the right and in front of the falls is steep and dangerous—best to avoid.

As you approach the falls from the north, you may look across the stream and see others arriving from the south. Here's an alternative approach for your next visit: during most of the late spring, summer, and fall, the Sundance chairlift takes hikers and mountain bikers from the base elevation of 6,100 feet to the summit at 7,150 feet in a matter of minutes (prices to ride: $11 adults, $9 children ages 6–12, $8 seniors age 65 and older, free for kids under age 6 with paying adult). From the summit, a pleasant downhill stroll leads to Stewart Falls at 6,800 feet, then back to Sundance. This loop hike is especially enjoyable in fall as the hillside blazes with autumn colors.

NEARBY ACTIVITIES

Nestled at the base of Mount Timpanogos and adjacent to Stewart Falls, **Sundance Resort (sundanceresort.com)** offers a diverse mountain-recreation experience year-round. Skiing, snowboarding, or cross-country skiing in winter and biking and hiking in summer all take place against a backdrop of breathtaking scenery. Lodging, fine dining, theater, and conference facilities make Sundance a favorite choice for an afternoon visit or an extended vacation.

49 BATTLE CREEK FALLS

KEY AT-A-GLANCE INFORMATION

LENGTH: 1.6 miles round-trip

ELEVATION GAIN: 450'

ELEVATION AT TRAILHEAD: 5,221'

CONFIGURATION: Out-and-back

DIFFICULTY: Easy

SCENERY: Deep-canyon waterfall and valley views

EXPOSURE: Mostly shaded

TRAFFIC: Moderate

TRAIL SURFACE: Dirt, rock

HIKING TIME: 45 minutes–1.5 hours

WATER REQUIREMENTS: 0.5 liter

SEASON: Year-round; minimal avalanche risk in winter

ACCESS: In Uinta-Wasatch-Cache National Forest. No fees or permits. Horses and mountain bikes also use this trail.

MAPS: USGS Orem, Trails Illustrated Uinta National Forest (701)

FACILITIES: Water and vault toilet near trailhead

DOGS: On leash

SPECIAL COMMENTS: Especially beautiful in autumn with colors and a trailbed of fallen leaves

GPS TRAILHEAD COORDINATES

N40° 21.789´ W111° 42.042´

IN BRIEF

A popular, family-friendly route along a creekbed in a deep canyon. The hike's payout: a 50-foot waterfall spraying down the side of a rock cliff.

DESCRIPTION

The Timpanogos massif, which dominates the eastern skyline of Utah County, has several canyons along its foothills that provide water to the towns below and access to the mountain's higher slopes. From the valley, you can most easily identify Battle Creek Canyon as the one immediately to the right (or south) of the G on the side of the mountain. Battle Creek supplies the water that fills the large tank and irrigates the orchards you pass on the way to the trailhead. In this area on February 28, 1849, a band of Ute Indians fought Captain John Scott and his men, pursuing Scott's party into the canyon.

Arriving at the parking area, walk toward the blue metal arch over the bridge that leads into Kiwanis Park. Find the trailhead by walking up the steep slope to your right, just a few feet before the bridge. Note the park's large

----

Directions ⟶

From Salt Lake City, go south on I-15 to Highland/Alpine (Exit 284). At the bottom of the off-ramp, turn left and take UT 92 east 7.4 miles toward the mouth of American Fork Canyon. As UT 92 enters the canyon, take UT 146 to the right and up the hill. Continue south 4.8 miles on UT 146 (Canyon Road) to 200 South in Pleasant Grove. Turn left onto 200 South and continue east 1.8 miles. As the pavement ends, continue another 0.3 mile up the wide dirt road, passing the large water tank on your way to the parking area next to Kiwanis Park.

Battle Creek Falls

Battle Creek Falls

89

water tank

P

Pleasant Grove

E. 200 S.

S. 1500 E.

UINTA-WASATCH-CACHE NATIONAL FOREST

N

| 0 | 0.1 | 0.2 | 0.3 miles |
| 0 | 0.1 | 0.2 | 0.3 kilometers |

6,000 ft.
5,800 ft.
5,600 ft.
5,400 ft.
5,200 ft.
5,000 ft.

Battle Creek Falls

Kiwanis Park

0.2 mi.   0.4 mi.   0.6 mi.   0.8 mi.

Battle Creek Falls

picnic pavilion, drinking water, and vault toilet, all under the shade of giant cottonwood trees. As the trail climbs the hillside, it soon joins a jeep road on the right.

Don't expect to see any water in the creekbed to your left. Because the water is diverted into underground pipes just up the canyon, it remains dry throughout the year. At 0.3 mile, you'll see a water-diversion basin where Battle Creek begins its life underground. Beyond this diversion basin, follow the tumbling creek another 0.2 mile and cross to the north side of the creek over a sturdy wooden footbridge.

After it crosses the bridge, the trail steepens considerably. Shards of shale from the cliffs above cover the trail's dirt base. Still, the trail provides sure footing. Within about 100 feet after you cross the bridge, the falls appear. About 50 feet before the falls, the trail divides. The right spur descends to the base of the falls, and the main trail to the left leads to the top.

A natural spring feeds Battle Creek, augmented by snowmelt. So while the falls' spray becomes heaviest in spring, the creek and the falls are perennial. Battle Creek Falls serves as a popular escape from summer's heat, with visitors enjoying the cooling spray near its base. The water falls gently enough that even young children can safely walk and play under the main channel of water as it bounces off the rock wall. Local adventurers often rappel down the falls in summer.

The trail leading to the top of the falls continues up the canyon and joins the Great Western Trail, which surrounds much of Mount Timpanogos and connects all the canyon trails on Timpanogos's western slopes.

At the lower elevations, below the falls, the vegetation consists of Gambel oak, sage, and cottonwoods. Conifers and aspens grow at higher elevations near the falls and above. You'll often spot pinyon jays, but scrub jays—while common— prove to be a bit more elusive.

Along the way, you're likely to see more people than animals. Families out for a day hike will find the trail suitable for children, while young couples and older adults can get some exercise just minutes from the neighborhoods in the valley below.

NEARBY ACTIVITIES

The U.S. Forest Service's **Pleasant Grove Ranger Station** (801-785-3563) is on the way to the trailhead at 390 N. 100 East (UT 146). The office offers maps and publications about recreation in Uinta-Wasatch-Cache National Forest.

50 PROVO RIVER PARKWAY

KEY AT-A-GLANCE INFORMATION

LENGTH: 15 miles one-way

ELEVATION GAIN: –702' (from Vivian Park to Utah Lake)

ELEVATION: 5,200' (Vivian Park trailhead), 4,498' (Utah Lake trailhead)

CONFIGURATION: One-way or out-and-back

DIFFICULTY: Easy

SCENERY: Deep canyon, mountain streams, waterfalls, towering peaks, pastures, wetlands

EXPOSURE: Partially shaded

TRAFFIC: Busy

TRAIL SURFACE: Paved

HIKING TIME: Varies

WATER REQUIREMENTS: 1 liter; drinking fountains (plus parks, restaurants, and convenience stores) along trail

SEASON: Year-round

ACCESS: No fees or permits

MAPS: USGS Bridal Veil Falls, Orem, Provo

FACILITIES: Restrooms, water, phone at trailhead and throughout hike

DOGS: On leash

SPECIAL COMMENTS: Check for avalanche risk November 1–March 31.

GPS TRAILHEAD COORDINATES

Vivian Park Trailhead:
N40° 21.327´ W111° 34.448´
Utah Lake Trailhead:
N40° 14.277´ W111° 43.922´

IN BRIEF

The Provo River Parkway is a community treasure, connecting residents with the river, mountains, waterfalls, parks, shopping, work, and Provo's history. As the parkway follows the course of the river, you're constantly exposed to the life of the river—trout fishing, waterfowl, and riparian plants. Take the trail in bite-size pieces and enjoy.

DESCRIPTION

The Provo River Parkway stretches from a deep mountain canyon through shopping centers, business parks, and neighborhoods to the shores of Utah Lake. Along its course, the trail passes through a national forest, 2 county parks, 14 city parks, and a state park.

While it's certainly possible to walk the trail from top to bottom, or vice versa, most choose to enter the parkway from one of dozens of access points and enjoy the scenic array found within just a mile or two in either direction. Officially designated as a nonmotorized multiuse trail, the parkway is widely used by families, seniors, and students as Provo's most popular venue for outdoor recreation and exercise.

On any given day you can see hundreds of people on the trail. But think of it as a highly social trail—not a crowded one. Inline skaters, skateboarders, kids on scooters, babies in strollers, cyclists, runners, and walkers all coexist happily, with pedestrians enjoying the right of way.

The most scenic section of the trail may be the upper 5 miles, from Vivian Park to the mouth of Provo Canyon (the intersection of US 189 and Orem 800 North). In addition to these two locations, you can enter the trail at

Provo River Parkway

MOUNT TIMPANOGOS WILDERNESS AREA

South Fork Provo River

Vivian Park Trailhead

Bridal Veil Falls

NUNNS PARK

BRIDAL VEIL FALLS PARK

UINTA-WASATCH-CACHE NATIONAL FOREST

Provo

Canyon Mouth Parking

189

N. University Avenue

89

Orem

52

15

S. Geneva Road

89

114

15

Utah Lake Trailhead

Utah Lake

3 miles
3 kilometers

5,400 ft.
5,200 ft.
5,000 ft.
4,800 ft.
4,600 ft.
4,400 ft.

Vivian Park

Orem 800 North (Mile 5)

Utah Lake

5 mi.   10 mi.   15 mi.

Directions ————————————————————————————→

VIVIAN PARK TRAILHEAD: From Salt Lake City, go south on I-15 to Orem 800 North (Exit 272). At the bottom of the off-ramp, turn left and proceed east 3.7 miles on 800 North (UT 52) toward the mouth of Provo Canyon. Take the left ramp onto East Provo Canyon Road (US 189). Go 5.8 miles to Vivian Park. Turn right on South Fork Road. Cross the railroad tracks and enter the parking area.

UTAH LAKE TRAILHEAD: From Salt Lake City, take I-15 south to Provo/Center Street/Airport (Exit 265). Turn right onto Center Street (UT 114) and continue west 2.5 miles to North 4200 West. Turn right and continue 200 feet to the parking area, on the right.

In addition to these starting and ending trailheads, an additional 15 official trailheads with public parking provide easy trail access.

----

many points in between, including Nunns Park, Canyon Glen, Mount Timpanogos Park, and Canyon View Park. These access points also offer drinking water and restroom facilities, plus tables and grates for a picnic after the hike.

Within this section, the trail and the river flow together, never more than 20 feet apart and always within view and earshot of each other. The steep canyon walls and wooded canyon floor offer abundant shade. You'll have multiple opportunities to stop and dangle your feet in the water or watch fly-fishermen try to snag a trophy cutthroat or rainbow trout.

Among the many scenic highlights in Provo Canyon, Bridal Veil Falls is a perennial crowd-pleaser. At 607 feet, this double cataract is the highest waterfall in Utah. In the spring and early summer, the water sprays onto the trail and hikers play in the runoff. In winter, the frozen falls and the Stairway to Heaven seepage to the right of the falls provide some of Utah's favorite ice-climbing routes. From Nunns Park or Bridal Veil Falls Park, the falls are just a 10-minute walk.

About 100 feet downstream from Bridal Veil Falls is a display of old mining equipment in front of an abandoned mine entrance, a reminder of the mining operations that played such an important role in the canyon's development. Another 100 yards downstream at Nunns Park are the remnants of an early hydroelectric plant built in 1897. At the time, the plant produced almost three times the voltage of any existing line in the nation and powered mining operations 32 miles to the west.

Throughout Provo Canyon you're likely to see raptors circling above, while belted kingfishers and yellow warblers flit along the riverbanks. Young children always seem fascinated by the snake grass (or horsetails), a tall, dark-green, tubular grass growing along the banks.

The lower section of the trail, from Geneva Road to Utah Lake, is every bit as beautiful as the Provo Canyon section, but in a very different way. You might even think you're on a different river in another state. As the river approaches the lake, it widens and slows. Whitewater kayaks are the upriver conveyance of choice, while below it's canoes or rowboats.

In the final 2.5 miles of the trail, the river meanders through a tunnel of mature cottonwoods. On the trail's north side are protected pastures frequented by egrets and warblers. To the south, the river and marshy lowlands host ducks, geese, and a wide variety of migrating waterfowl. You can easily reach this wetlands section of the trail from Fort Utah Park, Oxbow Park, or Utah Lake State Park.

Between the canyon and the wetlands, the Provo River Parkway passes through neighborhoods and busy shopping centers, and under city streets and I-15. While this center section of the trail lacks the scenic beauty of the canyon and the rural appeal of the lowlands, it does offer a safe, convenient place for local residents to get outdoors and enjoy a walk along the river.

Although cyclists have a 15-mph speed limit and pedestrians enjoy the right of way, you still need to keep to the right or in the marked pedestrian lane and be on guard for cyclists approaching from behind. Access to the swift-moving river is never fenced or protected, so supervise young children carefully at all times. Throughout its 15-mile length, the trail is entirely paved and well marked. The almost imperceptible incline rarely varies, so you can enter at any point for a leisurely stroll or a vigorous workout.

NEARBY ACTIVITIES

If just walking along the banks isn't enough excitement for you, try rafting the Provo River. **High Country Rafting** at Frazier Park (just downstream from Vivian Park) offers exciting trips down the Provo River on mild (Class II) whitewater during the summer season. Trips down the river last about 2 hours and can be guided or unguided in a raft, tube, or kayak. Call 801-224-2500 or visit **highcountry rafting.com** for information and reservations.

51 BIG SPRINGS HOLLOW

KEY AT-A-GLANCE INFORMATION

LENGTH: 5 miles round-trip

ELEVATION GAIN: 554'

ELEVATION AT TRAILHEAD: 5,796'

CONFIGURATION: Out-and-back with loop

DIFFICULTY: Easy

SCENERY: Mountain views to the west and natural springs with perennial flow. Trail follows creek.

EXPOSURE: Mostly shaded

TRAFFIC: Moderate. Go midweek for more solitude.

TRAIL SURFACE: Dirt, moderate incline

HIKING TIME: 1.5–2.5 hours

WATER REQUIREMENTS: Carry 1 liter; water at springs is generally safe at source.

SEASON: Year-round. Ideal snowshoe or ungroomed cross-country-skiing trail in winter.

ACCESS: No fees or permits

MAPS: USGS Bridal Veil Falls, Trails Illustrated Uinta National Forest (701)

FACILITIES: Restrooms and water fountain in park (closed/shut off in winter)

DOGS: On leash

SPECIAL COMMENTS: Some areas may become boggy in spring. Negligible avalanche risk in winter.

GPS TRAILHEAD COORDINATES

N40° 19.938´ W111° 31.456´

IN BRIEF

From the city park trailhead, a steady ascent follows a small creek through a broad valley to Big Springs, a natural spring flowing from the mountainside. Mountain views, abundant valley vegetation, and frequent wildlife sightings make this a popular and accessible family adventure.

DESCRIPTION

Take everything you ever imagined about a city park—the crowds, passing cars, cityscapes. Now throw it all out the window. True, the land in Big Springs Hollow is largely owned by the city of Provo, and the trailhead starts in the city-park parking lot. But in less than a minute, the parking lot is out of sight and you're suddenly enveloped in a secluded mountain valley in search of the natural springs that feed the meandering creek at your side.

The main trail follows the south side of this wide, slope-sided valley as the creek crisscrosses the trail several times. Sturdy wooden bridges span all the major creek crossings. For the first 0.7 mile, the trail makes a moderate but steady climb, finally arriving at a knoll

----

Directions _____→

From Salt Lake City, go south on I-15 to Orem 800 North (Exit 272). At the bottom of the off-ramp, turn left and proceed east 3.7 miles on 800 North (UT 52) toward the mouth of Provo Canyon. Take the left ramp onto East Provo Canyon Road (US 189). Go 5.8 miles to Vivian Park. Turn right on South Fork Road. Cross over railroad tracks, pass Vivian Park, and continue up South Fork Canyon for 3 miles. Turn right to enter Big Springs Park. Continue to the upper-level parking area, where you'll find the trailhead in the lot's southwest corner.

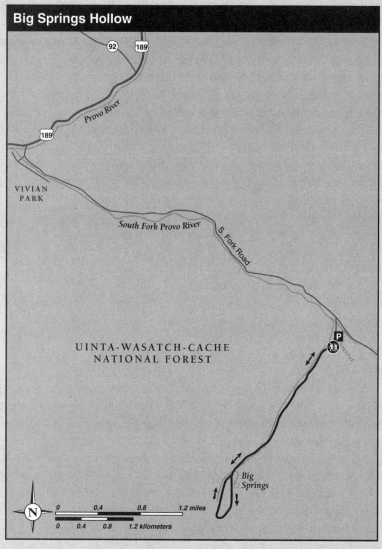

Big Springs Hollow

92 189

Provo River

189

VIVIAN
PARK

South Fork Provo River

S. Fork Road

UINTA-WASATCH-CACHE
NATIONAL FOREST

P

*Big
Springs*

N

| 0 | 0.4 | 0.8 | 1.2 miles |

| 0 | 0.4 | 0.8 | 1.2 kilometers |

7,500 ft.

7,000 ft.

6,500 ft.

Big Springs

6,000 ft.

5,500 ft.

5,000 ft.

0.5 mi.   1 mi.   1.5 mi.   2 mi.   2.5 mi.

where the terrain flattens a bit. After a brief 0.1 mile of level trail, the slope steepens and the ascent returns. Mountain views of Cascade Peak and the back side of the Wasatch Front remain ahead of you to the west for most of the hike.

Throughout the hike, quaking aspen and bigtooth maple provide most of the shade, while thickets of poplar, river birch, and willow cluster near the creek.

Following 30 minutes of steady hiking and immediately after a creek crossing, you'll come to a sign marking a fork in the trail. To the left, another 0.5 mile ahead, is Big Springs. The fork to the right leads to the Cascade Saddle at 4.1 miles. Just after you take the trail's left fork, you'll cross the creek on a wooden bridge. By the time you reach the sign, you'll have gained nearly 500 feet in elevation since leaving the trailhead.

From this point on to the springs, the trail steers closer to the south side of the valley. Along this slope, stands of aspen give way to Douglas-fir and the trail soon rises above the creek, although it's never more than about 50 feet away and always within earshot.

Another 0.3 mile beyond the first sign, you'll come to a second sign at the junction of the Cascade Springs Trail. Turn right at this T-junction and continue toward Big Springs, just 0.2 mile ahead.

The trail is designated as a nonmotorized multiuse trail, meaning it's used by horse riders, mountain bikers, hikers, and—in winter—skiers and snowshoers. They all seem to get along pretty well. Hikers still predominate in summer and snowshoers in winter. The gentle side slopes of the valley make avalanche risk negligible, and there is no history or visible evidence of avalanches in the area around the trail.

As you approach Big Springs, the woods deepen and become more coniferous, with some scrub-oak underbrush. The last 0.1 mile before arriving at Big Springs proves the steepest section of trail, but not steep enough to require switchbacking or any special treatment.

Cascade Springs flows from several release points on the mountainside and fans down the slope to the left of the trail. A small water-diversion culvert to the right of the trail directs some of the water toward the main creek channel. Big Springs marks the high elevation point of the hike, at 6,350 feet. The water from Big Springs flows down to South Fork Creek and into the Provo River. Big Springs is the largest of many small springs, seeps, and willow bogs throughout the canyon. Some of the area's springs have been Provo drinking-water sources for more than 60 years.

From Big Springs, follow the trail down the slope to the right and cross another wooden bridge. About 0.2 mile past Big Springs, the trail merges with the Cascade Trail. This junction represents the turnaround point on the loop. Take a hard right and follow the Cascade Trail east and back to the trailhead parking area. Continuing west on the trail will lead to the Cascade Mountain Saddle and to Rock Canyon Campground. From this trail junction, ambitious hikers could access a much larger network of trails and actually return to Provo city on foot over the Cascade Mountain Saddle and down Rock Canyon.

On the return, the north side of the loop passes a permanent site used by the Provo School District as an environmental camp for elementary students in June. You'll find a drinking fountain with chlorinated water here during the summer. The trail passes wet and dry grassy meadows with lupine, clover, violets, and mustards. A local rancher still cuts and harvests a spread of alfalfa here.

Throughout the year, hikers can expect to see deer, rabbits, and the occasional moose. Mountain lions roam the hillsides, and you'll frequently see their tracks in the winter snow, although you're unlikely to actually see this elusive species. Wild turkeys, ruffed grouse, and many songbirds can be spotted in the summer. During one recent summer, a survey of butterflies reported 60 different species in Big Springs Hollow between March and September, with western skippers and western bluetails being the most common.

Weather can change rapidly on the eastern slopes of the Wasatch. Particularly in the fall and winter, once the sun sets or the clouds roll in afternoon temperatures can drop quickly.

After returning to the parking area, you'll find the tables, fire grates, and covered group sites inviting spots for relaxing or enjoying an afternoon picnic or cookout. With their higher elevations, mountain shade, and cooler temperatures, South Fork Canyon and Big Springs Hollow are a popular summer retreat.

NEARBY ACTIVITIES

Utah County residents use **Provo Canyon** as a year-round playground. Anglers, river runners, and hikers can find lots to keep them busy through most of the year. In the depths of winter, you'll often spot ice climbers ascending the frozen overspray of Bridal Veil Falls. Vivian Park, at the mouth of South Fork Canyon, is a popular picnic area and serves as the starting point for the historic Heber Valley Railway. The billowing steam engine takes tourists up Provo Canyon from Vivian Park to Soldier Hollow and the Heber Valley. Call 435-654-5601 or visit **heber valleyrr.org** for schedules, special events, and information.

52 BUFFALO PEAK

KEY AT-A-GLANCE INFORMATION

LENGTH: 1 mile round-trip

ELEVATION GAIN: 287'

ELEVATION AT TRAILHEAD: 7,738'

CONFIGURATION: Out-and-back

DIFFICULTY: Easy

SCENERY: Sweeping views of Utah Valley and surrounding peaks

EXPOSURE: Partially shaded

TRAFFIC: Light

TRAIL SURFACE: Dirt with shale near summit

HIKING TIME: 30 minutes–1 hour

WATER REQUIREMENTS: 0.5 liter; no water on or near trail

SEASON: Late spring–early fall

ACCESS: No fees or permits. The gate near the top of Squaw Peak Road is closed late October–mid-May (depending on weather).

MAPS: USGS Bridal Veil Falls

FACILITIES: No facilities at trailhead or on trail

DOGS: Permitted

SPECIAL COMMENTS: You'll enjoy this trail most on a clear day in late spring with wildflowers in bloom, or in early fall as trees start to turn colors at high elevations. Bring a camera or binoculars.

GPS TRAILHEAD COORDINATES

N40° 16.973´ W111° 36.313´

IN BRIEF

If you're after a great view with very little effort, Buffalo Peak is the easiest, most accessible summit on the Wasatch Front. Within minutes of the trailhead, you're overlooking Utah Valley from an elevation of more than 8,000 feet. And you'll likely have the trail and the summit to yourself.

DESCRIPTION

If you were to fill Provo's LaVell Edwards Stadium to capacity with 65,000 local residents, then ask them where Buffalo Peak is, you might find only a handful who could point it out. From the valley floor, Buffalo Peak is a fairly nondescript rounded knoll, north of the more striking Squaw Peak and west of Cascade Peak. It doesn't appear in the USGS Geographic Names Information System database, yet at 8,025 feet in elevation, it's higher than many popular peaks on the Wasatch Front. It's unfortunate that this peak has gone unrecognized for so long, because Buffalo Peak stands

----

Directions

From Salt Lake City, go south on I-15 to Orem 800 North (Exit 272). At the bottom of the off-ramp, turn left and proceed east 3.7 miles on 800 North (UT 52) toward the mouth of Provo Canyon. Take the left ramp onto East Provo Canyon Road (US 189). Drive 1.8 miles to Squaw Peak Road and turn right. Continue 4 miles up Squaw Peak Road to the intersection of Squaw Peak Road and Forest Service Road 027. Turn left on FR 027 toward Hope Campground. At 0.4 mile the pavement ends. Continue another 2.9 miles on the dirt road to the unmarked trailhead, with a log-rail fence on the right and a fire-prevention sign on the left side of the road.

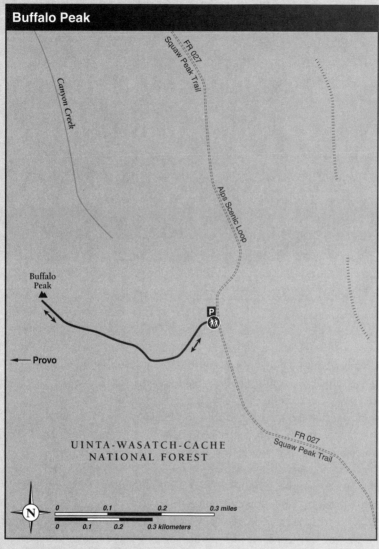

Buffalo Peak

Canyon Creek

FR 027
Squaw Peak Trail

Alps Scenic Loop

Buffalo
Peak

P

Provo

FR 027
Squaw Peak Trail

UINTA-WASATCH-CACHE
NATIONAL FOREST

N

0   0.1   0.2   0.3 miles
0   0.1   0.2   0.3 kilometers

8,200 ft.
8,100 ft.
8,000 ft.   Buffalo Peak
7,900 ft.
7,800 ft.
7,700 ft.
        0.1 mi.   0.2 mi.   0.3 mi.   0.4 mi.   0.5 mi.

Buffalo Peak, with Cascade Peak as a backdrop

out as one of the best short hikes in Utah County. You'll enjoy an easy stroll to some dazzling views, all against the solitude of a mountainous backdrop.

At the unmarked trailhead you can park at the side of the dirt road and easily crawl over or under the log fence. You almost feel like you're sneaking onto private property, but the hike lies within the Uinta-Wasatch-Cache National Forest. From the fence, continue up the trail through a grassy meadow sprinkled in spring with violet-blue larkspur and yellow bursts of mulesear wyethia.

Deer and cougars visit these dry mountain slopes infrequently. Ground squirrels prove to be more-active inhabitants, and with some luck you'll see a black-headed grosbeak or mountain chickadee.

At 100 yards, the trail leaves the grassy clearing and enters a clump of aspen and oak. As the trail continues its gradual ascent, you come to some early partial views of Utah Valley below, with the trail laid out clearly ahead of you. At 0.3 mile, a trail forks to the right, but your summit lies directly ahead. Soon the trail steepens, as the path is sprinkled with chips of shale. The final 0.1-mile push to the summit requires you to negotiate a steep slope of shale and dirt.

After just 0.5 mile of walking from the trailhead, you come to the Buffalo Peak summit, a balding shale outcrop crowned with curly-leaf mountain mahogany, maple, and Gambel oak. In autumn, these hillsides take on the look of a patchwork quilt with lemon-colored aspen, fiery maples, and golden oaks. Take in the excellent views stretching from Mount Nebo on the south to the Salt Lake Valley on the north. You overlook Squaw Peak (elevation 7,877 feet) directly to the south, with the summit of Cascade Peak (elevation 10,760 feet) directly to the east, just 1.6 miles away as the crow flies.

NEARBY ACTIVITIES

Utah Valley's traditional lovers' lane, the **Squaw Peak Overlook** is a mandatory stop on your way to or from Buffalo Peak. At an elevation of 6,707 feet, it's the perfect drive-to viewpoint for day or evening views of the valley below. From the intersection at the top of Squaw Peak Road and FR 027, turn right and continue 0.3 mile to the overlook parking area.

53 SQUAW PEAK

 KEY AT-A-GLANCE INFORMATION

LENGTH: 7 miles round-trip

ELEVATION GAIN: 2,709'

ELEVATION AT TRAILHEAD: 5,167'

CONFIGURATION: Out-and-back

DIFFICULTY: Moderate

SCENERY: Rock formations, canyon, hillside forest, mountain meadow, panoramic views at summit

EXPOSURE: Mostly shaded

TRAFFIC: Busy

TRAIL SURFACE: Paved for first 0.4 mile, rocky for next 1.2 miles, then dirt to summit

HIKING TIME: 3.5–5 hours

WATER REQUIREMENTS: 1.5–2 liters, depending on heat

SEASON: Spring, summer, fall

ACCESS: Year-round access; no fees or permits

MAPS: USGS Bridal Veil Falls

FACILITIES: Restrooms and water at trailhead

DOGS: On leash

SPECIAL COMMENTS: The mouth of Rock Canyon provides a great place to watch or participate in rock climbing.

GPS TRAILHEAD COORDINATES

N40° 15.879´ W111° 37.791´

IN BRIEF

One of the most popular summit hikes in Utah County, the climb to the top of Squaw Peak offers memorable highlights such as the dramatic rock walls of Rock Canyon, a climb through a wooded hillside, and panoramic views from the summit. You'll particularly enjoy the hike after the aspens have leafed out in the spring or when they turn a fiery yellow in the fall.

DESCRIPTION

At just 7,876 feet in elevation, Squaw Peak is considered one of the lesser peaks of the Wasatch Range, but it cuts an unmistakable profile as it rises above the craggy cliffs on Provo's east bench. It's also one of the most deservedly popular day hikes on the Wasatch Front.

The trail to the summit can be broken into three distinctive chunks: the canyon approach, the hillside ascent, and the summit stretch. Each section has its own characteristic appeal, and all combine to form a challenging hike offering varied features and highlights. The first 1.5 miles follow the Rock Canyon

----

Directions

The trail begins at the mouth of Rock Canyon, behind the LDS Temple in Provo. From Salt Lake City, take I-15 south to Orem/University Parkway (Exit 269). Exit to the left and continue east 5 miles on University Parkway (UT 265) to 900 East in Provo. Turn left on 900 East and continue north 0.4 mile, then turn right on Temple View Drive. Continue up Temple View Drive to East 2300 North. Turn right on East 2300 North and continue east 0.4 mile to the trailhead parking lot, straight ahead.

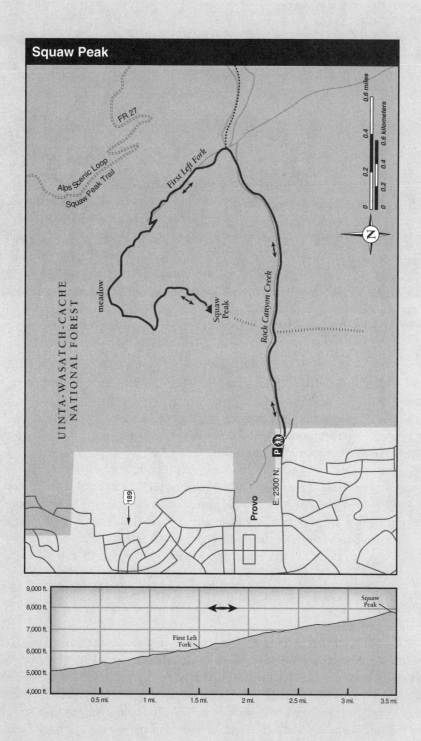

Squaw Peak

FR 27

Alps Scenic Loop

Squaw Peak Trail

First Left Fork

Rock Canyon Creek

meadow

Squaw Peak

UINTA-WASATCH-CACHE
NATIONAL FOREST

189

Provo

E. 2300 N.

P

0.6 miles
0.4
0.2
0

0.6 kilometers
0.4
0.2
0

N

9,000 ft.
8,000 ft.
7,000 ft.
6,000 ft.
5,000 ft.
4,000 ft.

Squaw
Peak

First Left
Fork

0.5 mi.   1 mi.   1.5 mi.   2 mi.   2.5 mi.   3 mi.   3.5 mi.

Hikers take in the views from Squaw Peak's summit.

Trail (#060) eastward up Rock Canyon. Then the route turns north onto the Squaw Peak Trail to the summit.

From the large trailhead parking lot, the trail is paved for the first 0.4 mile as it leads toward the mouth of Rock Canyon through a covering of sage and Gambel oak. After a few hundred feet, the asphalt road forks. The forks (one asphalt, the other surfaced with roadbed) soon rejoin, but bear right if you want to stay on the surfaced road. Easy access to some great routes makes Rock Canyon one of the most popular rock-climbing areas in Utah County. The first rock face on your right is the popular Black Rose wall, with Red Slab to the right. Just after the pavement ends, the trail passes through a metal gate and leads to a small cove of climbing faces on the right called The Kitchen.

Beyond the gate, the rocky trail steadily ascends the dry creekbed and passes through a wide canyon. At 0.5 mile past the gate, you'll come to the first of five wooden footbridges crossing the creek. At this point, with the higher elevation, conifers first appear.

On the north side of the creek, at 1.1 miles past the Kitchen gate, you'll come to a brown plastic flap-pole Forest Service sign indicating a trail up the hillside draw to the left, known as the First Left Fork. This begins the second chunk of the hike—the hillside ascent—which begins at an elevation of 6,100 feet. After 1.1 miles of steady climbing, you'll reach a meadow at 7,240 feet. No switchbacks offer relief. But the trail surface is well worn and smooth, and the setting is a thick forest of Gambel oaks and quaking aspens. The climb is steep, the experience rewarding.

In the hillside forest you may spot deer and small cats. Mountain lions and even bears make an occasional appearance in Rock Canyon, but they are rare. You're much more likely to see mountain chickadees—which often nest and breed above 8,000 feet—along the hillside trail in spring and summer.

Crossing the high meadow begins the third chunk of the hike—the summit stretch. The trail curves to the left along the southern rim of the meadow through a stand of aspens. Leaving the meadow, the path now heads south toward the summit ahead. You'll climb steadily, but the trail is not quite as steep as the hillside section behind you.

On the way to the summit, the oak cover becomes shorter and juniper dots the hillside. Here you'll first glimpse both the valley to the east and the higher peaks to the west (which are snowcapped well into June). Deer often graze above the meadow; you may even spot them at or near the summit.

Generally, Utah Valley to the west provides the most popular view from the summit. You may feel like you're looking straight down at the trail below, and, interestingly, the trail near the mouth of the canyon is about 2,500 feet to the south, with a vertical drop of 2,700 feet. On most days, you can see Mount Nebo to the south and Mount Timpanogos to the north.

As long as you're taking in the panorama, don't forget the peaks behind you to the east. Cascade Mountain (10,908 feet) is the rounded peak with the striated face to the northeast. Lightning Peak is the triangular (11,044) peak in the background to the east, and Provo Peak (11,068) is in the forefront to the southeast. Squaw Peak's summit offers plenty of large, flat rocks that make the perfect table for a summer picnic with a view.

NEARBY ACTIVITIES

With its steep ascents, Squaw Peak supplies a good workout in spring, summer, and fall. During the winter, you may be relegated to Brigham Young University's indoor jogging track in the **Smith Fieldhouse.** Near the corner of 1060 North and 150 East in Provo, the fieldhouse also hosts BYU volleyball games and other events.

54   Y MOUNTAIN

KEY AT-A-GLANCE INFORMATION

LENGTH: 2.2 miles round-trip

ELEVATION GAIN: 1,102'

ELEVATION AT TRAILHEAD: 5,164'

CONFIGURATION: Out-and-back

DIFFICULTY: Moderate

SCENERY: Continuous views of Utah Valley below

EXPOSURE: No shade

TRAFFIC: Busy

TRAIL SURFACE: Compacted dirt and rock

HIKING TIME: 1–2 hours

WATER REQUIREMENTS: 1 liter. Water at trailhead; none on trail.

SEASON: Year-round, day or night; trail may have snow in winter

ACCESS: Ample free parking at trailhead

MAPS: USGS Provo

FACILITIES: Restrooms at trailhead

DOGS: On leash

SPECIAL COMMENTS: A popular trail, well worn by local families and students. Short but steep.

GPS TRAILHEAD COORDINATES

N40° 14.690´ W111° 37.632´

IN BRIEF

The immense concrete letter Y on the mountainside directly east of the Brigham Young University campus in Provo is visible for miles around Utah Valley. The trail to the Y is a series of a dozen switchbacks offering splendid views of the valley along the way. It's a popular workout or training hike.

DESCRIPTION

At 380 feet high and 130 feet wide, the white Y on Y Mountain is the largest collegiate symbol in the United States—even larger than the HOLLYWOOD sign in the Los Angeles hills. While it can be seen throughout much of Utah Valley, it's also a great place from which to view the valley itself.

The trailhead also provides public access to the Bonneville Shoreline Trail and to the extended Y Mountain Trail for those hikers wanting to continue beyond the Y and on to the summit.

Directions ⟶

The trail begins in the foothills directly east of the BYU campus in Provo. From Salt Lake City, take I-15 south to Orem/University Parkway (Exit 269). Exit to the left and continue east 5 miles on University Parkway (UT 265) to 900 East in Provo. Turn right on 900 East and continue south 0.8 mile to 820 North. Turn left onto 820 North and continue east. After 0.5 mile, 820 East veers left and becomes Oakmont Lane. Continue 0.1 mile along Oakmont Lane to Oakcliff Drive. Turn right on Oakcliff Drive and ascend 0.1 mile to 1450 East. Turn right and continue 0.1 mile to Terrace Drive. Turn right and follow Terrace Drive 0.1 mile. Before you reach the end of the cul-de-sac, turn left onto 940 North, which leads 0.3 mile up the hill to the trailhead parking lot.

Y Mountain

UINTA-WASATCH-CACHE
NATIONAL FOREST

Terrace Drive

Oak Cliff Drive

Oakmont Lane

Provo

E. 820 N.

Arlington Heights Drive

0.3 miles
0.2
0.1
0
0.3 kilometers
0.2
0.1
0

7,500 ft.
7,000 ft.
6,500 ft.
6,000 ft.
5,500 ft.
5,000 ft.

"Y"

0.25 mi.   0.5 mi.   0.75 mi.   1 mi.   1.1 mi.

The trail to the Y

The wide, well-marked trail is a series of ten steep switchbacks leading to the bottom of the Y, plus four more for those continuing to the top of the Y. The trail is on private land owned by BYU up to the second switchback, after which you enter Uinta-Wasatch-Cache National Forest. The city of Provo maintains the trail-head parking area.

Because the trail ascends more than 1,000 feet in just over a mile, this is a popular workout hike, with many residents climbing the path several times a week. No bikes are allowed on the trail, so hikers can move at their own pace and not feel chased. Throughout the hike you have views of the valley below, with no trees to block the view—or the afternoon sun. In the heat of summer you'll see why this hike is popular in the early morning, before the sun crests over the peaks above.

The first two switchbacks are the longest and cover nearly 0.4 mile. For those climbing to the top of the Y, the sign at the fifth switchback marks the halfway point for both distance and elevation gain. The tenth switchback is a good rest stop where you can study the photographic panel identifying local peaks and land-marks in the valley below. From this point it's another 0.1 mile to the bottom of the Y. Taking just four more short switchbacks 0.3 mile up the mountain leads you to the top of the Y.

Y Mountain juts out from the western slopes of the Wasatch Range to deliver sweeping views of Utah Valley, from Mount Nebo in the south to Lone Peak in the north. Across Utah Lake to the northwest are the Oquirrh Mountains, and the

Lake Mountains rise up from the western shores of Utah Lake. The freestanding mountain on the southwest shore of Utah Lake is West Mountain.

The Y was first placed on the mountain in 1906 and enhanced in 1907 with a layer of rock. In 1911 it was enlarged to its present size and made into a block Y with a base of rock, sand, and concrete. Viewed straight-on from the air, the letter appears elongated, but it was designed that way so it would look normal from the valley floor. In order to reduce both ongoing maintenance costs and the risk of falling, hikers are encouraged not to climb on the surface of the Y.

Scrubby Gambel oak, sage, and grasses cover the mountain slope. Because the trail is steep and lacks dense vegetation, hikers must stay on the path to mini-mize erosion. While the trail is steep, it's safe even for young children, with most drop-offs protected by log-rail fencing.

Along the way, chukars frequently cross the trail from their nests in the brush. Magpies and jays appear year-round at lower elevations. Deer graze on the mountain slopes throughout the year, and bighorn sheep occasionally make their way down to the trail area.

Most hikers make the Y their destination and return the way they came up. If you have time, water, and energy to spare, the trail continues from the Y, head-ing south to Slide Canyon, then north to the summit of Y Mountain at 8,569 feet. It's another 3 miles to the summit (a total of 8 miles round-trip from the trail-head). For those going to the summit, it's nice to know that the steepest part of the trail is all below the Y. If you go just to the Y, you've had a great workout with some well-earned views along the way.

NEARBY ACTIVITIES

The **Brigham Young University** campus sprawls below the trailhead. After you've hiked to the Y, a stop at the Creamery on Ninth for an ice-cream cone or a shake is a well-deserved guilty pleasure. The Wilkinson Center houses a large food court, the BYU Bookstore, and even a bowling alley on the lower level. The BYU Museum of Art showcases an exceptional permanent collection and plays host to world-class traveling exhibits. The Monte L. Bean Life Science Museum (645 E. 1430 North) houses a fascinating and extensive display of animal life. It's a fun place where both adults and children can view regional wildlife and big game from around the world.

West: Tooele County (Hikes 55 and 56)

55 Stansbury Island

Stansbury Island Trail

Great Salt Lake

80

196

80 **Burmester**

To Salt Lake City →

Burmester Road

138

Grantsville

UINTA-
WASATCH-CACHE
NATIONAL
FOREST

Stansbury Mountains

Mormon Trail

196

S. Willow Road

DESERET PEAK
WILDERNESS

56

Deseret
Peak

N

| 0 | 2 | 4 | 6 miles |
| 0 | 2 | 4 | 6 kilometers |

WEST
(TOOELE COUNTY)

55 STANSBURY ISLAND TRAIL

KEY AT-A-GLANCE INFORMATION

LENGTH: 9.5 miles

ELEVATION GAIN: 619'

ELEVATION AT TRAILHEAD: 4,275'

CONFIGURATION: Loop

DIFFICULTY: Moderate

SCENERY: Great Salt Lake, geology of Lake Bonneville shoreline

EXPOSURE: No shade

TRAFFIC: Light

TRAIL SURFACE: Dirt, rock

HIKING TIME: 3.5–4.5 hours

WATER REQUIREMENTS: 1–2 liters, depending on season; no water on trail

SEASON: Hikable year-round but best in early spring

ACCESS: No fees or permits. Trail is managed by the Bureau of Land Management and open to hikers, cyclists, and equestrians.

MAPS: USGS Corral Canyon, Plug Peak

FACILITIES: No restrooms or water at trailhead

DOGS: Permitted

SPECIAL COMMENTS: Driving to the trailhead, you'll pass salt-evaporation ponds. Morton, Cargill, and other salt companies extract about 2.5 million tons of salt from the lake annually.

GPS TRAILHEAD COORDINATES

N40° 48.377´ W112° 31.234´

IN BRIEF

Stansbury Island provides a fascinating glimpse into the geology and natural history of the Great Salt Lake. This loop hike gains all of its elevation in the first mile before following the ancient shoreline of a much larger lake. Solitude, salt, and sweeping lake views define the experience.

DESCRIPTION

When Jim Bridger first saw the Great Salt Lake on an expedition in the winter of 1823–24, he thought it was an arm of the Pacific Ocean. In reality, the Great Salt Lake is the remnant of Lake Bonneville, a much larger prehistoric freshwater lake that was the size of Lake Michigan and covered most of northern Utah. Unless you're armed with some knowledge of the ancient Bonneville shoreline, this could be a fairly mundane desert hike. Let's take a moment to review:

About 15,000 years ago, the elevation of Lake Bonneville was about 5,200 feet. This shoreline left a visible "bench," which is prominent along much of the Wasatch Front. Then, about 14,500 years ago, the lake washed away

----

Directions ———————→

From Salt Lake City, take I-80 west to Grantsville/UT 138 (Exit 84). Turn left onto the access road heading west. Continue on this road for 7.1 miles as it curves north onto Stansbury Island, becomes Stansbury Island Road, and heads north along the island's western shore. Turn right and follow a dirt road 0.2 mile to the BLM trailhead. (*Note:* If on the access road you come to a cattle grate followed by a NO TRESPASSING sign, you've gone too far north. Turn around and go back 0.4 mile to the dirt road leading to the trailhead.)

Stansbury Island Trail

Great Salt Lake

Stansbury Island

BOMBER CANYON

TABBYS CANYON

NO NAME CANYON

80

Great Salt Lake

N

| 0 | 0.3 | 0.6 | 0.9 miles |
| 0 | 0.3 | 0.6 | 0.9 kilometers |

5,200 ft.
5,000 ft.
4,800 ft.   Bench Trail
4,600 ft.
4,400 ft.
4,200 ft.

        2 mi.   4 mi.   6 mi.   8 mi.   9.5 mi.

Salt-evaporation ponds to the south, with Deseret Peak in the distance

a natural dam near Red Rock Pass in southeastern Idaho, which resulted in a cata-strophic flood, draining the lake to a much smaller size. Over the course of a year the Lake Bonneville shoreline dropped to a lower level, known as the Provo shore-line, which had an elevation of about 4,840 feet—380 feet lower than the earlier Bonneville shoreline. Stansbury Island provides the best-preserved and most visible example of the Provo shoreline. Our hike follows this shoreline around the southern end of the island as it winds along the level contour of several large canyons.

When Howard Stansbury, a government surveyor, first explored the island in 1849, water entirely surrounded it. Since then, the Great Salt Lake has retreated from its 1875 high-water level, leaving Stansbury Island as a peninsula. As you take the road to the trailhead, watch for the many migratory shorebirds found in the wetlands and pools at the south end of the lake. Once on the island, the shore-birds disappear, replaced by meadowlarks and other range and field birds.

From the trailhead, follow the trail to the south, across the alluvial plain and up a rocky slope. At 1.2 miles, you've arrived at the high elevation for the hike, just under 5,000 feet. After crossing the saddle you drop a little more than 100 feet in elevation, and the trail begins its 4-mile love affair with the Provo shore-line. As the contour of the shoreline enters canyons and rounds hillsides, the trail never gains or loses more than 10 feet in elevation. It sticks with the shoreline until making its final descent back to lake level.

The first canyon you skirt is the fairly small Bomber Canyon. At 1.8 miles you come around the bend to enter Tabbys Canyon, the largest of the canyons and one with dramatic views. After following the deep and clearly visible shoreline contour of Tabbys Canyon for 2.8 miles, you round the hillside to wide-open views of the Great Salt Lake and the Oquirrh Mountains to the east. To the south are the Stansbury Mountains and Deseret Peak. Geologically, Stansbury Island is actually a small northern extension of the Stansbury Mountains.

At 5.2 miles you'll find yourself at the head of No Name Canyon, on the southeast side of the island. At a fork in the trail, take the faint path to the right that descends the slope directly for 0.5 mile to a jeep road that loops back to the trailhead along the flat desert terrain just above lake level. Once you reach the dirt road, the Flexipole signs do a good job of guiding you back to the trailhead, although it's a pretty intuitive route. If you want to avoid hiking on jeep trails, you can leave a shuttle vehicle at the mouth of No Name Canyon and make this a one-way 6.4-mile hike.

Stansbury Island offers a field course in geology. Along the way you'll pass outcrops of shale, limestone, quartzite, and conglomerates that look for all the world like concrete—but they're not. The calcium carbonate deposits that form much of the Provo shoreline, known as tufa rock, were formed by precipitation from the high dissolved-calcium content of Lake Bonneville. You'll find tufa rock used in many early Utah homes in areas such as Bountiful and Pleasant Grove, which are near the Provo shoreline level.

Although the trail is hikable year-round, plan to visit in early spring, when the sheep grass is green and the sage and juniper are at their most aromatic. By mid-May, the range grasses dry and turn brown, and with no shade or water on the trail it can quickly become a hot desert hike.

With every step of the hike, you'll have great views of the Great Salt Lake and distant mountains. To the south you'll be looking down on the evaporation ponds used for the commercial production of salt. More than 4.5 billion tons of salt are dissolved and suspended in the Great Salt Lake, which has no outlet. About 2.2 million tons of salt enter the lake annually from surface and groundwater flow, while salt industries extract about 2.5 million tons of salt and other elements from the lake each year. As you look out over a lake that was once 1,000 feet deep, it's interesting to note that today the Great Salt Lake has a maximum depth of only 35 feet, with an average depth of just 14 feet. While no fish live in the lake, abundant brine shrimp serve as a food source for the millions of migratory birds that pass through the area every year.

NEARBY ACTIVITIES

Saltair, a resort on the shores of the Great Salt Lake, hosts concerts, events, and parties and features beach access and showers (435-243-7258; **thesaltair.com**). Built in 1893 by the Salt Lake and Los Angeles Railroad Company at a cost of more than $350,000, its pavilion was destroyed by fire in 1971 and rebuilt in 1981. To the west of Saltair is **Great Salt Lake Marina State Park,** with a well-developed marina, electricity, and a pumpout station.

56 DESERET PEAK

KEY AT-A-GLANCE INFORMATION

LENGTH: 8.5 miles

ELEVATION GAIN: 3,603'

ELEVATION AT TRAILHEAD: 7,428'

CONFIGURATION: Loop

DIFFICULTY: Hard

SCENERY: Wooded approach, high-mountain terrain, excellent views

EXPOSURE: Mostly shaded below 10,000', fully exposed above 10,000'

TRAFFIC: Light

TRAIL SURFACE: Dirt, rock

HIKING TIME: 5–7 hours

WATER REQUIREMENTS: 2 liters; water in streams can be purified.

SEASON: Late spring, summer, early fall

ACCESS: No fees or permits

MAPS: USGS Deseret Peak East, Deseret Peak West

FACILITIES: Restrooms at trailhead

DOGS: On leash

SPECIAL COMMENTS: Entire hike lies within the Deseret Peak Wilderness Area. Motorized vehicles and bicycles are prohibited.

GPS TRAILHEAD COORDINATES

N40° 28.978´ W112° 36.398´

IN BRIEF

At 11,031 feet, Deseret Peak is the highest point in Tooele County and the centerpiece of the Deseret Peak Wilderness Area. It's also a magnificent expanse of both semiarid and alpine scenery—glacial basins, mountain streams, woodland, and high meadows—rising from the middle of the desert. This loop hike captures some of that surprising variety and affords views across the Bonneville Salt Flats and into Nevada.

DESCRIPTION

The Great Basin, which covers western Utah and most of Nevada, consists of dozens of north-to-south-trending mountain ranges and basins. Best known for their impact on local weather patterns and their jagged profile revealed with each sunset, the Oquirrh Mountains bound the Salt Lake Valley on the west. The Stansbury Mountains, which lie just to the west of the Oquirrhs and Tooele Valley, don't attract as much attention. Wasatch hikers rarely climb Deseret Peak, the jewel of the Stansbury Mountains. And that's a shame, since the area has so much to offer.

The drive to the trailhead captures the transformation from desert to mountain as the

Directions

From Salt Lake City, take I-80 west to Grantsville (Exit 84). From the exit, turn left to cross under I-80 and continue south 9.5 miles on UT 138 to Grantsville. Turn right on West Street (400 West) and continue 5 miles to South Willow Canyon (marked by a sign). Continue west 7.2 miles on South Willow Canyon Road to the Loop Campground. The last 4 miles of the road are unpaved. You'll find the trailhead at the top of the loop, to the right of the vault toilets.

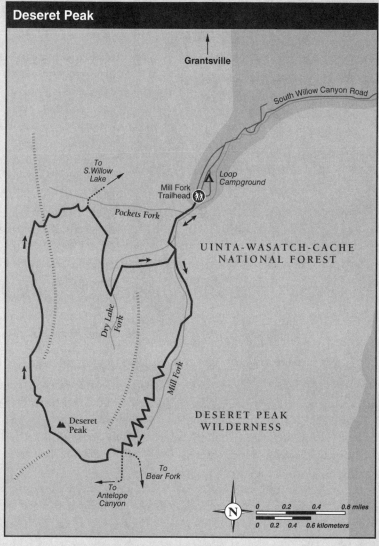

Deseret Peak

Grantsville

South Willow Canyon Road

To
S. Willow
Lake

Mill Fork
Trailhead

Loop
Campground

Pockets Fork

UINTA-WASATCH-CACHE
NATIONAL FOREST

Dry Lake
Fork

Mill Fork

Deseret
Peak

DESERET PEAK
WILDERNESS

To
Bear Fork

To
Antelope
Canyon

N

0   0.2   0.4   0.6 miles

0   0.2   0.4   0.6 kilometers

Deseret
Peak

Mill
Fork

Pockets
Fork

12,000 ft.
11,000 ft.
10,000 ft.
9,000 ft.
8,000 ft.
7,000 ft.

2 mi.   4 mi.   6 mi.   8.5 mi.

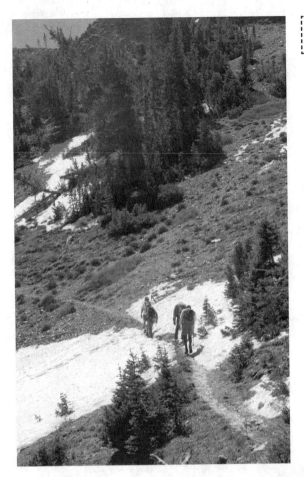

Deseret Peak's trails hold snow well into June.

road ascends an alluvial plain into the mouth of the canyon. You'll drive through two narrows with barely enough room for both the road and the stream to pass through the high rock walls rising above. Nearing the trailhead, you're likely to see wild turkeys and deer along the roadside. On its way to the trailhead, the road gains nearly 2,500 feet of elevation, giving hikers a good head start on the summit.

From the trailhead, a dense forest of aspen and conifers quickly immerses you. This section of the trail provides a vivid example of the aspen-to-conifer succession cycle. Aspen appear early in a woodland life cycle. Conifers, which initially are shaded and protected by aspen, eventually shade out the aspens. Many of the large, mature aspens have fallen in this area, while the conifers remain.

At 0.7 mile from the trailhead, you'll reach a stream crossing. Immediately after the crossing, the trail dips momentarily before coming to a sign and trail junction. Take the trail on the left to Deseret Peak. This junction marks the start of a clockwise loop that will take you up one drainage, along much of the Deseret Peak ridgeline to the summit, and then bring you back by way of another drainage.

At 1.1 miles from the trailhead, you'll enter the lower level of Mill Fork, a large glacial valley ringed by Douglas-fir. The trail leads to the top of a steep glacial bowl, gaining nearly 2,200 feet of elevation in 2.3 miles. After a series of switchbacks near the top of the bowl, you'll arrive at the ridge and enjoy your first views of the Great Basin to the west. On this ridge, at a four-way junction, a sign points the way to Bear Fork on the left, Antelope Canyon directly ahead, and Deseret Peak to your right. Take the trail to the right as it leads almost directly up a shadeless slope to a higher rocky ridge. The trail skirts some false summits before arriving at the true summit nearly a mile from the junction. Along the way, you'll gain an appreciation for the hardy limber pine and subalpine fir that survive a tortured existence at 11,000 feet. In late spring and summer, wildflowers line the rocky trail all the way to the summit.

You'll share the summit with cliff swallows as they swoop and dart around the rocky ledges. Because the Stansbury Mountains are an isolated, stand-alone range, Deseret Peak has nothing nearby to block the view. On a clear day—which in summer is nearly every day—you can see Pilot Peak in Nevada more than 60 miles to the northwest. Mount Nebo is visible to the southeast.

Most Wasatch peak-baggers never see the Bonneville Salt Flats from a summit, but they're easily viewed from Deseret Peak. This 6,000-square-mile bed of salt, known as "the flattest place on earth," is the site of numerous land speed records.

To make the return loop, continue north as you descend along the summit ridge. After 0.3 mile, the trail drops well below the ridge on the west side. When you've hiked 1.5 miles from the summit, the trail makes a sharp turn to the right and continues its descent of the east side of the ridge in a series of short switch-backs. At 2.2 miles from the summit, having descended Pockets Fork, you'll come to a sign pointing to South Willow Lake to the left and the Loop Campground, your return route, to the right. As the trail sweeps along a bowl, making a gradual descent, you'll have picture-postcard views of the ridge above and to the west. Soon you enter the familiar aspen–spruce woodland that leads back to the stream-crossing junction and down to the trailhead.

Not many peaks allow hikers to do a loop and take in such a variety of eco-systems and rough wilderness terrain by means of a well-marked, easy-to-follow trail. A Deseret Peak loop offers hikers abundant scenery, a real appreciation for the immense size of the wilderness area, and a sense of how much is available to explore.

NEARBY ACTIVITIES

Tooele Valley is home to the **Deseret Peak Complex,** a multipurpose public recreation venue that features one of Utah's largest swimming pools, complete with a water-slide and wading area, as well as professionally designed and maintained tracks for motocross, BMX, ATV, and horse racing. Within the complex you'll also find soccer fields, softball diamonds, pitch-and-putt golf, playgrounds, an archery park, indoor and outdoor arenas, pavilions, and two museums. For general and special-events information, call 435-843-4020 or visit **deseretpeakcomplex.com.**

East: Uintas/Summit County (Hikes 57–60)

Kamas Lake

To Evanston, WY

Picturesque Lake

Butterfly Lake

Butterfly Campground

57

Bud Lake

UINTA-WASATCH-CACHE NATIONAL FOREST

58

Pass Lake

150

Bonnie Lake

Blythe Lake

Mirror Lake Campground

Bald Mountain

Moosehorn Campground

Moosehorn Lake

HIGH UINTAS WILDERNESS

59

150

Fehr Lake

60

Bald Mountain Pass

N

To Kamas & Salt Lake City

Murdock Mountain

80 **40**

0   4   8   12 miles

0   4   8   12 kilometers

EAST
(UINTAS/SUMMIT COUNTY)

57 NATURALIST BASIN

KEY AT-A-GLANCE INFORMATION

LENGTH: 12–18 miles round-trip

ELEVATION GAIN: 996' (low elevation: on trail, near Scudder Lake, 9,950'; high elevation: Faxon Lake, 10,946')

ELEVATION AT TRAILHEAD: 10,376'

CONFIGURATION: Out-and-back with loop and spur options

DIFFICULTY: Hard

SCENERY: Lakes and ponds, spruce forests, wildflowers, surrounding mountains

EXPOSURE: Mostly shaded to Naturalist Basin, fully exposed on upper basin above tree line

TRAFFIC: Moderate

TRAIL SURFACE: Dirt, some rock

HIKING TIME: 6–10 hours

WATER REQUIREMENTS: 2 liters; water in lakes and streams can be purified.

SEASON: Summer

ACCESS: Within the Uinta-Wasatch-Cache National Forest fee-recreation area (see page 4). Pick up a recreation pass at the Kamas Ranger Station or at one of the self-service fee stations along the Mirror Lake Scenic Byway.

MAPS: USGS Hayden Peak, Trails Illustrated High Uintas Wilderness (711)

FACILITIES: Restrooms, picnic tables, and drinking water at trailhead

DOGS: Permitted

GPS TRAILHEAD COORDINATES

N40° 43.325´ W110° 51.842´

IN BRIEF

A rolling trail through a basin of woods, meadows, and scenic lakes, almost entirely above 10,000 feet in elevation. While the complete loop with spur trails to nearby lakes can cover more than 20 miles, it can easily be adapted to a shorter 12-mile hike. But the gentle, flowing nature of the trail makes you want to go on to the next lake or meadow.

DESCRIPTION

The beauty of the Uinta Mountains is as likely to be found in its complex network of basins and drainages as in its quartzite peaks. Here, unlike the canyons of the Wasatch, you're never quite sure of where the water comes from or the direction in which it flows. Naturalist Basin, which lies east of the Mirror Lake Scenic Byway, generally flows south into the Duchesne River. But the rolling, meandering nature of the trail never makes that clearly visible to the hiker.

Naturalist Basin sits to the south of Mount Agassiz, named for the great Swiss-American naturalist Louis Agassiz. Most of the lakes in the basin were named after Agassiz's students at Harvard and Cornell, many of whom went on to become prominent scientists and naturalists in their own right: David Starr

----

Directions

From Salt Lake City, take I-80 east to Silver Creek Junction/US 40 (Exit 146). Take US 40 east 3.4 miles to UT 248 (Exit 4). At the end of the off-ramp, turn left and continue on UT 248 for 11.4 miles to South Main Street (UT) in Kamas. Turn left on South Main Street and go north for two blocks, then turn right on Center Street (UT 150). Continue 34.2 miles on UT 150 (just past Mile Marker 34) to the Hayden Pass–Highline trailhead.

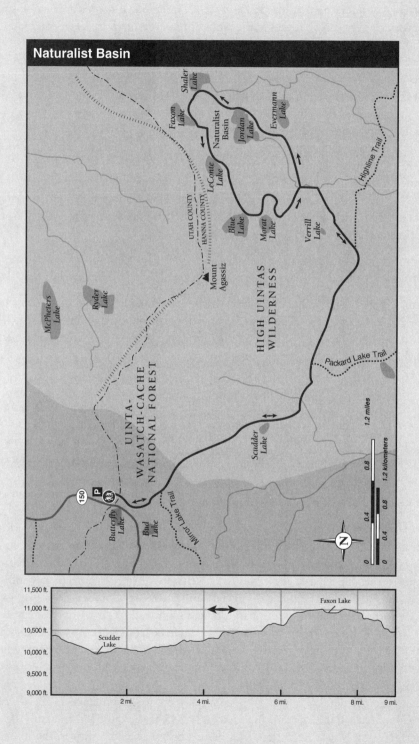

Naturalist Basin

Shaler Lake

Faxon Lake

Naturalist Basin

Evermann Lake

Jordan Lake

LeConte Lake

UTAH COUNTY

HANNA COUNTY

Blue Lake

Morat Lake

Verrill Lake

Mount Agassiz

Highline Trail

HIGH UINTAS WILDERNESS

McPheters Lake

Ryder Lake

Packard Lake Trail

UINTA-WASATCH-CACHE NATIONAL FOREST

Scudder Lake

Mirror Lake Trail

150

P

Butterfly Lake

Bud Lake

1.2 miles

1.2 kilometers

0.8

0.8

0.4

0.4

0

0

N

11,500 ft.

11,000 ft.

10,500 ft.

10,000 ft.

9,500 ft.

9,000 ft.

Scudder Lake

Faxon Lake

2 mi.   4 mi.   6 mi.   8 mi.   9 mi.

Jordan, Nathaniel Shaler, Joseph LeConte, Charles Walcott, and Alpheus Packard. Agassiz's legacy can be found in the names of many American species and natural landmarks.

Naturalist Basin is accessed from the Highline Trail (#083), which crosses the Uintas from east to west. Almost all of the trail's 60-mile length is above 10,000 feet in elevation, and much of it is above tree line. The large trailhead parking area to the south serves hikers, while the parking area to the north has loading ramps and facilities for horses and stock.

From the trailhead, the trail descends 200 feet in elevation through a forest of Engelmann spruce to a junction with the Mirror Lake Trail at 0.7 mile. Continue on the Highline Trail to the southeast. At about 2 miles from the trailhead, you'll pass Scudder Lake to the south and continue another mile before arriving at a junction with the Packard Lake Trail (#059), which leads south on a 1.4-mile optional spur to Wilder, Wyman, and Packard lakes.

In these woods you're likely to see woodpeckers and pine grosbeaks. One species you're not likely to see is the bark beetle, an insect about the size of a piece of rice; but you'll certainly see the damage it's done to trees throughout the Uintas. Bark beetles are native insects that kill individual trees but do not threaten the entire tree species. Healthy trees normally produce enough defensive pitch to flush out the attacking beetles. But when trees are stressed and weakened, they're unable to produce sufficient amounts of pitch. In recent years, more trees have been killed by bark beetles than by forest fires.

Continuing along the Highline Trail for another 1.2 miles, you'll arrive at a marked junction where the trail forks. Go left and to the north into Naturalist Basin. (The Highline Trail continues to the right.) The trail makes a gradual ascent for about a mile into Naturalist Basin, eventually crossing a stream and arriving at an open meadow with a backdrop of Uinta cliffs and 12,428-foot Mount Agassiz to the northwest.

At this point, you've hiked a little more than 5 miles from the trailhead and you're at the edge of Naturalist Basin. Jordan Lake (elevation 10,625 feet), a popular fishing destination, is another mile up the trail to the northeast. Morat Lakes (10,757 feet), about a mile to the northwest, also attract the anglers. But if you got off to an early start and still have plenty of energy, consider taking the loop to the upper basin. Few hikers take this loop, since it ascends beyond the tree line into a more remote and rugged alpine ecosystem, but it is certainly worth the effort. To reach this upper basin, take a faint trail leading from the east side of Jordan Lake up a rocky slope to Shaler Lake (10,920 feet). As you ascend just 300 feet of elevation, you move from a subalpine to an alpine ecosystem, where everything changes. You'll find different animals, birds, wildflowers, and trees as you explore this high-alpine shelf.

From Shaler Lake, the loop continues on to Faxon Lake (10,946 feet), LeConte Lake (10,925 feet), Blue Lake (10,945 feet), and Morat Lakes (10,757 feet). Passing Morat Lakes, the trail descends 300 feet to return to the junction and stream crossing where you first entered Naturalist Basin. From here you can pick up the trail that returns you to the Highline Trail and on to the trailhead, another 5 miles to the west.

Naturalist Basin is popular but never really busy. The trail is well traveled but never crowded. It's relaxing, meandering, and therapeutic, and in spite of its long distance and high elevation it's suitable for hikers of various skill levels. For the most part the route is intuitive, but you should take a GPS, or a map and compass, and be proficient in their use.

NEARBY ACTIVITIES

The **Samak Smoke House** is a favorite one-stop shopping destination for visitors to the Mirror Lake Scenic Byway. Just 2 miles east of Kamas at 1937 Mirror Lake Highway, the country store and restaurant is a convenient place to pick up your recreation pass and any provisions you might need for the hike. On the return trip, stop and try their famous jerky, and smoked salmon or trout. Shop for gifts and gourmet foods or dine out on the patio. For orders and information, call 435-783-4880 or shop online at **samaksmokehouse.com.**

58   LOFTY LAKE LOOP

KEY AT-A-GLANCE INFORMATION

LENGTH: 4.1 miles

ELEVATION GAIN: 920' (Reids Meadow to the pass east of Lofty Lake)

ELEVATION AT TRAILHEAD: 10,154'

CONFIGURATION: Loop

DIFFICULTY: Moderate

SCENERY: Alpine lakes, streams, meadows, mountains

EXPOSURE: Mostly shaded below 10,500', partially shaded above 10,500'

TRAFFIC: Moderate

TRAIL SURFACE: Dirt, rock

HIKING TIME: 3–4 hours

WATER REQUIREMENTS: 1–2 liters; water in lakes and streams can be purified.

SEASON: Summer

ACCESS: Within the Uinta-Wasatch-Cache National Forest fee-recreation area (see page 4). Pick up a recreation pass at the Kamas Ranger Station or at one of the self-service fee stations along the Mirror Lake Scenic Byway.

MAPS: USGS Mirror Lake, Trails Illustrated High Uintas Wilderness (711)

FACILITIES: Restroom at trailhead

DOGS: Permitted

SPECIAL COMMENTS: A section of trail passes through Camp Steiner, the highest-elevation Boy Scout camp in the United States.

GPS TRAILHEAD COORDINATES

N40° 42.848´ W110° 53.582´

IN BRIEF

Lofty Lake Loop has something for everyone—lakes, streams, deep woods, meadows, ridge routes, mountain passes, and scenic views—all within a convenient loop. There are a few steep ascents and descents, but they're never too long. Some route-finding and map-reading are required, but it's never too challenging. The hike is well suited to families and children capable of hiking 4 miles over varied and sometimes rugged terrain. The entire hike is above 10,000 feet in elevation, so be on guard for symptoms of altitude sickness.

DESCRIPTION

Lofty Lake Loop is the perfect introductory hike into all the scenic beauty that the Uinta Mountains have to offer. It's a loop hike (as you may have already guessed from its name), so you never retrace your route. New territory, surprises, and fresh sights wait around every corner.

The trail can be hiked in either direction, but the clockwise loop described here seems to be the general preference for several reasons: If you get an early start, the wildlife-viewing is likely to be better in the clockwise direction.

Directions

From Salt Lake City, take I-80 east to Silver Creek Junction/US 40 (Exit 146). Take US 40 east 3.4 miles to UT 248 (Exit 4). At the end of the off-ramp, turn left and continue 11.4 miles on UT 248 to South Main Street (UT 32) in Kamas. Turn left on South Main Street and go north for two blocks, then turn right on Center Street (UT 150). Continue 32 miles on UT 150 to the Pass Lake trailhead. Enter the large loop parking area, on the left (west) side of the road.

Lofty Lake Loop

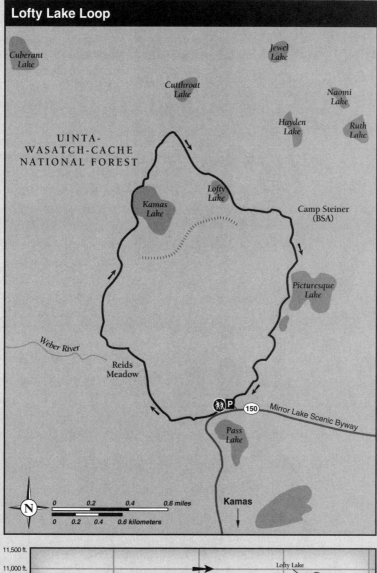

Cuberant Lake

Jewel Lake

Cutthroat Lake

Naomi Lake

Hayden Lake

Ruth Lake

UINTA-
WASATCH-CACHE
NATIONAL FOREST

Lofty Lake

Camp Steiner (BSA)

Kamas Lake

Picturesque Lake

Weber River

Reids Meadow

150 Mirror Lake Scenic Byway

Pass Lake

Kamas

N

| 0 | 0.2 | 0.4 | 0.6 miles |

| 0 | 0.2 | 0.4 | 0.6 kilometers |

11,500 ft.

11,000 ft.

Lofty Lake

Kamas Lake

10,500 ft.

Reids Meadow

10,000 ft.

9,500 ft.

9,000 ft.

1 mi.   2 mi.   3 mi.   4.1 mi.

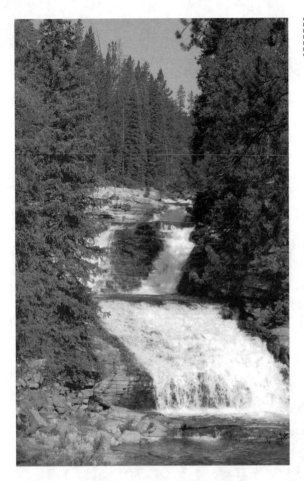

Provo River Falls (see Nearby
Activities, opposite page)

Also, the steepest sustained grade on the trail occurs as a descent near the end if done clockwise. The trail leading clockwise from the trailhead to Kamas Lake generally offers more solitude than the section from Lofty Lake back to the parking lot, which passes through the Boy Scout camp.

The trail starts near the restroom, at the southwest side of the parking lot, and ends just 100 feet away, on the north side of the lot. In addition to the Lofty Lake Trail, the trailhead serves the Weber River and Cuberant Lake trails. You'll know you're on the right trail when, 50 feet into the woods, you come to a sign directing you to Holiday Park (7 miles) and Cuberant Lake (3 miles).

At this sign, take the trail to Holiday Park and Cuberant Lake, to the right. At 0.3 mile you'll come to another fork, where you'll take the Cuberant Lake Trail to the right. You'll find occasional muddy surfaces along these lower sections of the trail. Wildflowers abound all along the trail, with Parry's primrose and alpine asters among the most common. Watch for Queen Anne's lace with its bursts of tiny white flowers; as a member of the carrot family, it has leaves that look just like carrot tops.

At 0.7 mile the trail crosses a small brook, then skirts the north side of a large, open, marshy area known as Reids Meadow. At 0.9 mile you leave the meadow by climbing a rocky slope to the north. At 1.2 miles from the trailhead, you come to another fork in the trail pointing to Cuberant Lake on the left and Kamas and Lofty lakes to the right. Continue up and to the right another 0.4 mile, along a rocky grade made up of chunky quartzite, and you'll soon arrive at a crest with Kamas Lake spread out immediately in front of you. The total distance from the trailhead to Kamas Lake is 1.6 miles. At this point you've descended just 150 feet from the trailhead to Reids Meadow, yet you've gained 520 feet in the climb up to Kamas Lake, at 10,520 feet in elevation.

Kamas Lake is a great place to rest before continuing on along the shore leading to a small man-made dam at the northwest end of the lake. From the dam, another steep, rocky ascent leads to a high meadow laced with small ponds and brooks and ringed with fir and spruce. Another steep ascent of a rocky slope leads to a crest above the meadow at an elevation of 10,700 feet and some dreamlike views of Teal, Cutthroat, and Jewel lakes to the north.

At this midpoint, just 0.5 mile beyond Kamas Lake, the trail begins to head south, crossing a high-alpine plateau sprinkled with wildflowers and Engelmann spruce. At the south end of the plateau you'll come to a small rise before dipping down to Lofty Lake, a shimmering jewel ringed by wildflowers. At an elevation of 10,840 feet, Lofty Lake is 2.5 miles from the starting trailhead.

Leading away from Lofty Lake, the trail rises and peaks at an elevation of 10,920 feet along a rock outcrop. Below is Scout Lake, easily identifiable by the boat dock, which serves the Scouts at Camp Steiner. From this high elevation point, it's just 1.4 miles back to the parking lot, and nearly all of it is downhill. The steepest part is right in front of you as you descend 520 feet in elevation down a rocky slope to the shores of Scout Lake.

The area around Picturesque Lake, which lies immediately south of Scout Lake, can be buggy and is the only portion of the trail where insect repellent may come in handy, especially in July. As with other hikes in the Uintas, afternoon thundershowers can appear quickly. If you see a storm gathering, find the quickest and safest route possible leading away from high, rocky elevations and back to the trailhead.

Leaving Picturesque Lake, the trail crosses a camp service road and continues along a gentle descent back to the parking area, completing the loop in 4.1 splendidly scenic miles.

NEARBY ACTIVITIES

For visitors on the Mirror Lake Scenic Byway, **Provo River Falls** is a must-see destination waterfall. It's actually a series of three distinct falls separated from each other by about 100 feet. From the parking and picnic area at the upper falls, take the paved trail to the second falls. An easy scramble leads to the river below the third falls. The falls parking area is on the left (west) side of the Mirror Lake Scenic Byway, just before Milepost 24.

59 FEHR LAKE TRAIL

KEY AT-A-GLANCE INFORMATION

LENGTH: 3.4 miles round-trip

ELEVATION GAIN: 472'

ELEVATION AT TRAILHEAD: 10,377'

CONFIGURATION: Out-and-back

DIFFICULTY: Easy

SCENERY: Lakes and ponds, spruce forests, wildflowers, mountains

EXPOSURE: Mostly shaded

TRAFFIC: Moderate

TRAIL SURFACE: Dirt, some rock

HIKING TIME: 1.5–3 hours

WATER REQUIREMENTS: 1 liter; water in lakes and streams can be purified.

SEASON: Late spring, summer, early fall

ACCESS: In the Uinta-Wasatch-Cache National Forest fee-recreation area (see page 4). Pick up a recreation pass at the Kamas Ranger Station or at one of the self-service fee stations along the Mirror Lake Scenic Byway.

MAPS: USGS Mirror Lake, Trails Illustrated High Uintas Wilderness (711)

FACILITIES: No facilities at trailhead; water and restrooms across the highway at Moosehorn Campground

DOGS: Permitted

SPECIAL COMMENTS: A rare mountain hike where the trailhead is at the higher elevation and each lake along the way takes you down the basin to a lower elevation. Save some energy for the hike out.

GPS TRAILHEAD COORDINATES

N40° 41.572´ W110° 53.503´

IN BRIEF

The Fehr Lake Trail descends along a route that skirts three alpine lakes and passes through woods and meadows, and along ponds and small streams. You can hike this trail as a short 1-mile stroll to Fehr Lake or continue to Shepard and Hoover lakes for a 3-mile round-trip walk—all in the shadow of Murdock Mountain to the southwest.

DESCRIPTION

This Uintas classic explores descending tiers of charming, jewel-like lakes. The lakes along the Fehr Lake Trail are part of the Duchesne River drainage, which eventually flows into the Green River and on to the Colorado River. The lakes to the south of the Bald Mountain summit flow into the Provo River and down to Utah Lake before terminating in the Great Salt Lake. This short hike can also be used as the starting point of an extended backpacking trip deep into the High Uintas Wilderness.

From the trailhead parking area, the trail departs southeast across a small wooden bridge over a marshy meadow. Soon the trail leaves the meadow and drops into a forest of fir and

----

Directions ———————————→

From Salt Lake City, take I-80 east to Silver Creek Junction/US 40 (Exit 146). Take US 40 east 3.4 miles to UT 248 (Exit 4). At the end of the off-ramp, turn left and continue 11.4 miles on UT 248 to South Main Street (UT 32) in Kamas. Turn left on South Main Street and go north for two blocks, then turn right on Center Street (UT 150). Continue 31 miles on UT 150 to a small, unpaved, unmarked parking area, on the right. It's just 100 yards south of the Moosehorn Campground, on the west side of the highway.

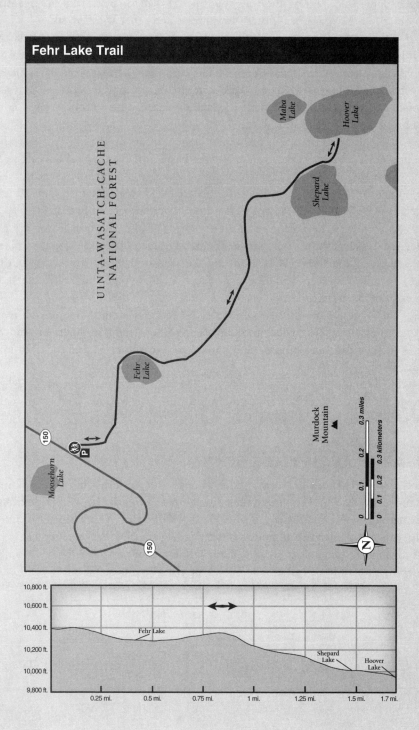

Fehr Lake Trail

Maba Lake

Hoover Lake

Shepard Lake

UINTA-WASATCH-CACHE
NATIONAL FOREST

Fehr Lake

Murdock Mountain

150

Moosehorn Lake

150

0.3 miles
0.3 kilometers

10,800 ft.
10,600 ft.
10,400 ft.
10,200 ft.
10,000 ft.
9,800 ft.

Fehr Lake

Shepard Lake

Hoover Lake

0.25 mi.   0.5 mi.   0.75 mi.   1 mi.   1.25 mi.   1.5 mi.   1.7 mi.

Engelmann spruce. Along the way you'll be treated to splashes of blue gentian, shooting star, elephant head, Parry's primrose, and other wildflowers.

At 0.2 mile you come to an unmarked junction, where you continue on the trail as it bears right. After crossing two more wooden bridges, you'll arrive at the shore of Fehr Lake (elevation 10,273 feet), which is less than 0.4 mile from the trailhead.

As you loop around Fehr Lake's eastern shore, the trail becomes faint as it crosses a low meadow and departs the lake. Insects can be a problem early in the season, so come prepared.

At 1 mile from the trailhead, a small pond appears on the left. The trail soon drops along a rocky channel as it enters the basin holding Shepard Lake. It's easy to lose the trail in this wooded stretch, but as long as you keep descending, you'll be on course. Soon, at 1.4 miles from the trailhead, you arrive at Shepard Lake (elevation 9,987 feet), a body of water about twice the size of Fehr Lake.

As you skirt the northeast shore of Shepard Lake, the trail leaves the lake and, just 100 feet east, rises to a small crest. Looking down the slope, you'll see the largest of the three lakes, Hoover Lake (elevation 9,220 feet), through the trees. Within 3 minutes you'll be at its shore. At this point you'll have hiked 1.7 miles from the trailhead.

The lakes are all stocked with fish, including arctic grayling, brook trout, brown trout, rainbow trout, and cutthroat trout. Common sights around the lakes include deer and moose, chipmunks, ground squirrels, and the occasional black bear.

High Uinta trails are notoriously winding and exceptionally scenic. Fehr Lake provides the perfect opportunity to dip into this lush wooded land of glistening alpine lakes.

NEARBY ACTIVITIES

As the **Mirror Lake Scenic Byway** passes through the western Uintas from Kamas, Utah, to Evanston, Wyoming, you'll find dozens of easily accessible developed campgrounds and inviting picnic areas for both day and overnight use. Additionally, you can choose from among hundreds of primitive backcountry campsites throughout the general forest area, many just a mile or two from the highway. For camping reservations, call 877-444-6777 or visit **recreation.gov.**

BALD MOUNTAIN

IN BRIEF

With a convenient trailhead and a well-groomed trail to the summit, Bald Mountain is an ideal climb, especially for children and inexperienced hikers who want to experience the thrill of climbing a high mountain summit. A National Recreation Trail recognized for its outstanding scenery, the Bald Mountain Trail offers wildflowers and breathtaking views of lakes and surrounding peaks in the High Uintas.

DESCRIPTION

The Uinta Mountains are part of a rare mountain range in the Western Hemisphere that runs east–west rather than north–south. At the western edge of the Uintas, Bald Mountain is a freestanding rounded peak that begs to be climbed. With a summit elevation of 11,943 feet, it's the most easily accessible high peak in Utah, higher than any peak in the Wasatch Range, and well worth climbing. Other Uinta peaks to the east are higher—including the highest point in Utah, 13,528-foot Kings Peak—but none are more suitable for a day hike.

Bald Mountain provides more than just bragging rights for making it to the top, though. It delivers spectacular summit views and gives

---

Directions

From Salt Lake City, take I-80 east to Silver Creek Junction/US 40 (Exit 146). Take US 40 east 3.4 miles to UT 248 (Exit 4). At the end of the off-ramp, turn left and continue 11.4 miles on UT 248 to South Main Street (UT 32) in Kamas. Turn left on South Main Street and go north for two blocks, then turn right on Center Street (UT 150). Continue 29 miles on UT 150 to the Bald Mountain trailhead–picnic area on your left. The trailhead is at the northwest corner of the large loop parking lot.

KEY AT-A-GLANCE INFORMATION

LENGTH: 3 miles round-trip

ELEVATION GAIN: 1,179'

ELEVATION AT TRAILHEAD: 10,764'

CONFIGURATION: Out-and-back

DIFFICULTY: Moderate

SCENERY: Wildflowers, high-alpine vegetation, exceptional Uintas views from summit

EXPOSURE: No shade

TRAFFIC: Busy

TRAIL SURFACE: Dirt, rock

HIKING TIME: 1.5–3 hours

WATER REQUIREMENTS: 1 liter; no water on trail

SEASON: Late spring, summer, early fall

ACCESS: Within the Uinta-Wasatch-Cache National Forest fee-recreation area (see page 4). Pick up a recreation pass at the Kamas Ranger Station or at one of the self-service fee stations along the Mirror Lake Scenic Byway.

MAPS: USGS Mirror Lake, Trails Illustrated High Uintas Wilderness (711)

FACILITIES: Restrooms and picnic area at trailhead; water at Mirror Lake Campground

DOGS: Permitted

SPECIAL COMMENTS: Bald Mountain is the highest peak in this book, yet it's one of the easiest to climb. It's normal to feel winded at this elevation, but watch for more-severe signs of altitude sickness, which include headache, nausea, vomiting, and dizziness.

GPS TRAILHEAD COORDINATES

N40° 41.348´ W110° 54.238´

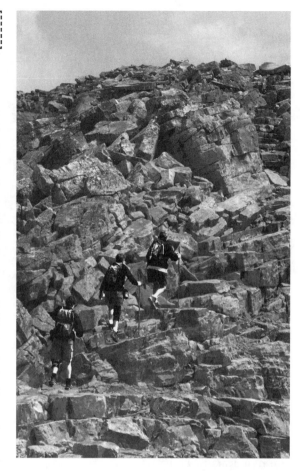

The rock staircase to the Bald Mountain summit

hikers the opportunity to move from a subalpine environment to a high-alpine zone while experiencing an amazing variety of wildflowers along the way. A herd of mountain goats inhabits the slopes of the mountain and can often be spotted on the plateau and above the tree line.

From the trailhead, at the edge of a meadow of lavender alpine aster, the trail passes through a small stand of spruce before hitting the rocky slope leading up the mountain. The trail, though unmarked, is well traveled and easy to follow.

At 0.6 mile, as the path approaches the tree line, you enter a large, rocky tundra plateau. The trail continues its ascent across this upper shelf, but at a more gentle gradient. As you reach the higher elevation, the alpine asters become noticeably smaller but just as vibrant. They are joined by moss campion, fiery Indian paintbrush, blue skypilot, and dozens of other wildflower species. At this high elevation, you'll find wildflowers you're unlikely to see in the Wasatch or in other areas of Utah. Subalpine fir makes its last appearance at about 11,400 feet, but the wildflowers continue to the summit.

At 0.9 mile the trail steepens to ascend a false summit. As you crest this mound, the true summit comes into view just 100 yards ahead. This last section of trail crosses a flat stretch of quartzite before climbing a short stairway of large, angular blocks. You'll encounter some big steps, but no scrambling is required.

Just 1.5 miles from the trailhead, you reach the expansive summit dome, with Reids Peak immediately to the northwest. The large, rounded peak to the east is Mount Agassiz (12,428 feet), while Hayden Peak (12,479 feet) is the jagged peak to the northeast. On a clear day you won't be able to count all of the lakes that lie in the basins below, but Moosehorn Lake lies immediately below,

Bald Mountain offers great views into the basins below.

between the highway and the eastern slopes of Bald Mountain. Mirror Lake is the larger lake to the north, on the east side of the highway.

Climb Bald Mountain early in the day. During the short summer season, afternoon thundershowers and lightning commonly occur in the Uintas. If such a storm appears to be brewing, you'd be wise to turn around and make a quick retreat to the parking area.

NEARBY ACTIVITIES

The **Kamas Ranger Station,** at 50 E. Center St. in Kamas (435-783-4338), makes an excellent starting point for a trip along the Mirror Lake Scenic Byway. The station has an interpretive center and offers an excellent assortment of books, maps, and resource materials for area trails, campgrounds, and activities.

APPENDIX A:
HIKING RETAILERS

BLACK DIAMOND
2092 E. 3900 South
Salt Lake City, UT 84124
801-278-0233
bdel.com

CABELA'S
2502 W. Grand Terrace Parkway
Lehi, UT 84043
801-766-2500
cabelas.com

HANSEN MOUNTAINEERING
1799 N. State St.
Orem, UT 84057
801-226-7498
hansenmountaineering.com

KIRKHAM'S OUTDOOR PRODUCTS
3125 S. State St.
Salt Lake City, UT 84115
801-486-4161
kirkhams.com

OUT N BACK
1797 S. State St.
Orem, UT 84097
801-224-0454
outnback.com

PATAGONIA
2292 S. Highland Drive
Salt Lake City, UT 84106
801-466-2226
patagonia.com

RECREATION OUTLET
recreationoutlet.com
615 E. State Road
American Fork, UT 84003
801-763-7722

3160 S. State St.
Salt Lake City, UT 84115
801-484-4800

2324 Washington Blvd.
Ogden, UT 84401
801-409-9994

REI
3285 E. 3300 South
Salt Lake City, UT 84109
801-486-2100
rei.com/stores/19

230 W. 10600 South, Suite 1700
Sandy, UT 84070
801-501-0850
rei.com/stores/81

SPORTSMAN'S WAREHOUSE
sportsmanswarehouse.com
165 W. 7200 South
Midvale, UT 84047
801-567-1000

1075 S. University Ave.
Provo, UT 84601
801-818-2000

1137 W. Riverdale Road
Riverdale, UT 84405
801-334-4000

APPENDIX B: HIKING CLUBS AND TRAIL ORGANIZATIONS

MOUNTAIN TRAILS FOUNDATION
P.O. Box 754
Park City, UT 84060
435-649-6839
mountaintrails.org

OUTDOORS UNLIMITED
Brigham Young University
1151 Wilkinson Student Center
Provo, UT 84602
801-422-2708
outdoors.byu.edu

SERAC MOUNTAINEERING CLUB
P.O. Box 1997
Orem, UT 84059
801-226-7498
seracclub.org

SHERYL'S OUTDOOR ADVENTURE CLUB
Sheryl McGlochlin, Director
Salt Lake City, UT
801-278-5313
liveandthrive.com

SIERRA CLUB, OGDEN GROUP
P.O. Box 1821
Ogden, UT 84402
utah.sierraclub.org/ogden

SIERRA CLUB, UTAH CHAPTER
2159 S. 700 East, Suite 210
Salt Lake City, UT 84106
801-467-9297
utah.sierraclub.org

UNIVERSITY OF UTAH OUTDOOR RECREATION PROGRAM
2140 E. Red Butte Road, Building 650
Salt Lake City, UT 84112
801-581-8516
utah.edu/campusrec

UTAH VALLEY UNIVERSITY OUTDOOR ADVENTURE CENTER
800 W. University Parkway, SC103H
Orem, UT 84058
801-863-7052
uvu.edu/oac

WASATCH MOUNTAIN CLUB
1390 S. 1100 East, Suite 103
Salt Lake City, UT 84105
801-463-9842
wasatchmountainclub.org

WEBER PATHWAYS
P.O. Box 972
Ogden, UT 84402
801-393-2304
weberpathways.org

WEBER STATE UNIVERSITY WILDERNESS RECREATION CENTER
4022 Taylor Ave.
Ogden, UT 84408
801-626-6373
weber.edu/wrc

APPENDIX C: GLOSSARY
OF SALT LAKE CITY–AREA
HIKING TERMS

Alpine Relating to mountains; often descriptive of plants, animals, and scenery found in mountainous regions.

Alpine zone Life zone found in regions above 11,500 feet; characterized by arctic-alpine tundra.

Avalanche A mass of snow, ice, and accompanying debris sliding down a mountain or over a cliff.

Berm A natural or man-made raised bank of earth that forms a low ridge.

Bonneville Shoreline, or Bench The geologic features visible at the 5,090-foot level on the mountains surrounding Salt Lake City. These deposits were left by the shoreline of ancient Lake Bonneville 15,000 years ago.

Boulder-hopping Hiking that involves walking and sometimes jumping across sections with large rocks.

Bowl A large depression left in the earth by a retreating glacier, often part of a cirque.

Bushwhack To clear a path through thick woods or undergrowth where no trail exists.

Cairn A stack of rocks created as a trail marker. Hikers often construct cairns to mark the way on faint trails.

Canopy A layer formed by the leaves and branches of the forest's tallest trees.

Cirque A deep-walled, glacier-carved basin on a mountain usually forming the blunt upper end of a valley.

Conifer Trees and shrubs that are typically cone-bearing and evergreen. In Utah, common conifers are spruce, fir, pine, and juniper.

Couloir A steep mountainside chute or gully that often retains snow late in the season.

Drainage An area (basin) generally bounded by ridges or slopes, encompassing a watershed.

Exposure Vulnerability; used to describe the potential for physical harm in the event of a fall.

Forb A broad-leafed plant other than grass, often found growing in fields and meadows.

Glacier A large body of ice moving down a slope or mountain.

Glissade To slide in a standing or sitting position down a snow-covered slope without using skis.

Knife-edge A mountain ridge, often close to the summit, characterized by a narrow passage and slopes that drop sharply on both sides.

Krummholz Trees and other wooded vegetation found near tree line that have been twisted and stunted by wind and severe weather.

Massif A compact portion of a mountain range containing one or more summits. Mount Timpanogos, for example, is a massif within the larger Wasatch range.

Montane zone Life zone found at elevations from 8,000 to 9,500 feet and characterized by aspen and Douglas-fir.

Moraine The rocks and soil carried and deposited by a glacier.

Outcrop The exposed part of a rock formation that can be seen above the ground.

Riparian Along or near a stream or river.

Route-finding Techniques of navigating in a backcountry or wilderness setting without using GPS, compass, or maps.

Saddle A ridge between two peaks.

Scrambling A type of climbing that does not entail the use of ropes; instead, hands and legs are used to provide propulsion and balance.

Scree Debris consisting of small loose rocks, usually fist-size or smaller.

Side canyon A tributary or branch of a larger canyon. Broads Fork and Mineral Fork, for example, are side canyons of Big Cottonwood.

Snowfield An expanse of snow cover that can either be permanent or last well beyond the winter season. The accumulation above Emerald Lake on Mount Timpanogos, for instance, is considered a permanent snowfield.

Subalpine zone Life zone found at elevations from 9,500 feet to tree line (about 11,000 feet) and characterized by spruce forests.

Switchback A zigzagging trail up the side of a steep slope or mountain. Allows for a more gradual and less strenuous ascent.

Talus A sloping mass of rock debris at the base of a cliff.

Tarn A mountain lake formed by a glacier.

Technical climbing Rock or mountain climbing involving the use of ropes and protective equipment.

Transition zone The foothills at an elevation of 5,500–8,000 feet, characterized by oak and maple shrublands.

Traverse A section of trail that moves across a slope or ridge in a horizontal direction.

Tree line (timberline) The elevation where the trees end and subalpine or alpine vegetation begins. The elevation of tree line varies with latitude and climate. In northern Utah, the tree line is around 11,000 feet.

Tundra The treeless vegetation found in high-alpine and arctic terrain, consisting of lichens, mosses, grasses, and low shrubs.

Watershed The land area that drains water into a river system or other body of water.

INDEX

Check out this great title from
Wilderness Press!

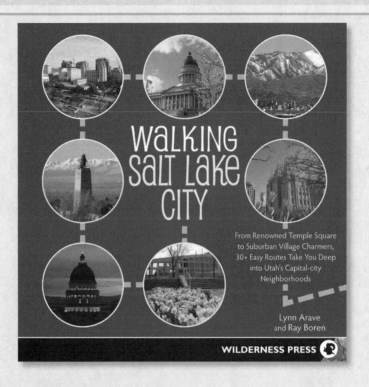

Walking Salt Lake City

By Lynn Arave and Ray Boren
ISBN: 978-0-89997-692-1
$17.95

7x7, paperback

Walking Salt Lake City is a time-traveling guide to Salt Lake City's past and to its vibrant present. Written by Utah natives, it presents rambles of every kind. The 30+ tours explore the city's downtown, which is experiencing an invigorating renaissance; Temple Square, world headquarters of the Latter-day Saints Church; Capitol Hill; character-filled neighborhoods like the Avenues and "15th and 15th"; and semirural surprises near and within the bustling city, from Memory Grove and City Creek Canyon, a stone's throw from metropolitan skyscrapers, to tucked-away and nearly forgotten Miller Bird Preserve and the appropriately named Hidden Hollow.